COMMUNICATION SKILLS FOR THE

Healthcare Professional

LAURIE KELLY McCORRY, Ph.D.

Dean of Science, Engineering and Health Programs
Bunker Hill Community College
Boston, Massachusetts

JEFF MASON, M.F.A.

Associate Dean of Academic Affairs
Bay State College
Boston, Massachusetts

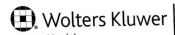 Wolters Kluwer | Lippincott Williams & Wilkins
Health
Philadelphia • Baltimore • New York • London
Buenos Aires • Hong Kong • Sydney • Tokyo

Acquisitions Editor: David B. Troy
Product Manager: John Larkin
Marketing Manager: Allison Powell
Designer: Steve Druding
Compositor: Aptara, Inc.

First Edition

351 West Camden Street   Two Commerce Square
Baltimore, MD 21201   2001 Market Street
                                          Philadelphia, PA 19103

Printed in The People's Republic of China

20 19 18 17 16 15 14 13 12 11 10

Library of Congress Cataloging-in-Publication Data

McCorry, Laurie Kelly, 1959-
   Communication skills for the healthcare professional / Laurie Kelly
McCorry, Jeff Mason. – 1st ed.
      p. ; cm.
   Includes bibliographical references and index.
   ISBN 978-1-58255-814-1 (alk. paper)
   1. Communication in medicine. I. Mason, Jeff, 1961- II. Title.
   [DNLM: 1. Communication–Problems and Exercises. 2. Professional-Patient Relations–Problems
and Exercises. 3. Allied Health Personnel—Problems and Exercises. W 18.2]
   R118.M395 2011
   610.69′6—dc22

                                                          2010043254

DISCLAIMER

To purchase additional copies of this book, call our customer service department at **(800) 638-3030** or fax orders to **(301) 223-2320**. International customers should call **(301) 223-2300**.

Visit Lippincott Williams & Wilkins on the Internet: **http://www.lww.com.** Lippincott Williams & Wilkins customer service representatives are available from 8:30 am to 6:00 pm, EST.

To Tat, ∞ × 9   —LKM

In Memory of Debra Viti, M.D.   —SJM

Today, poor communication is the single most common reason for patient complaints against healthcare professionals. One cannot overstate the importance of having good communication skills in any of the allied health professions. The healthcare provider who has strong communication skills will always be more effective in helping patients. Good communication has been shown to improve patient satisfaction, patient compliance, and patient health outcomes. Recent studies have indicated that many patients value the communication skills of their healthcare provider even higher than the provider's technical skills. Senior clinicians and managers across the healthcare industry routinely attribute their success to their having been effective communicators.

Students preparing for careers in health care must not only master the science and clinical skills necessary to providing quality patient care, they must also become strong communicators. *Communication Skills for the Healthcare Professional* helps meet this need by providing allied health students with a comprehensive yet compact guide to learning essential communication skills.

Intended to supplement the clinical coursework students complete in the first one to two years of all allied health programs, the book uses a broad range of examples, role plays, and scenarios from virtually every healthcare field, giving both instructors and students the ability to use it as a manual to master any area-specific communication skill. Each chapter provides students with objective and short-answer questions to test comprehension of the material, as well as more complex clinical applications, encouraging students to develop the critical thinking skills they will need every day as professionals in the healthcare industry.

Organized into three main sections outlining basic communication principles and their uses in clinical and administrative settings, *Communication Skills for the Healthcare Professional* is easy to reference and can serve as a guide long after the course in which the student first encounters it. This compact and user-friendly format makes for a book that can accompany the student during the first clinical internship, or even into the first full-time job.

Acknowledgments

We would like to express our warmest thanks to the following people:

At East Boston Neighborhood Health Center: Geraldine Alquinta, Kaddour Fradj, Marlene Garcia, Maria Garcia Soneira, Marcela Gil, Garry Lenescat, Genevieve Majano, Silvia Mendoza, Nadia Nabat, Gloria Nieves, Ginna Ospina, Wandaly Pellicier, Lidia Quijano, Monica Ramirez, Beatriz Ramos, Angelica Sabouni, Jeymi Severino, and Yesley Villatoro helped us to better understand how to make this a more useful book to allied health students. As the first class to use this text during its development, they showed patience, largeness of spirit, and sound knowledge in each of their disciplines.

At Bay State College: Bill Carroll, Ph.D.; Rosana Darang, M.D.; Janice Meckstroth, M.Ed.; Donnalee Shain, P.T., M.S., D.P.T.; at Boston University: Susan Blau, M.A.; and at the Joseph M. Smith Community Health Center: Ann E. White, R.N., M.S., who all generously shared their time and expertise in helping to make this a better book.

In South Boston: Kit Kelly, for coming back.

Contents

PART II:

Clinical Communication Skills   55

CHAPTER
4

Professional Communication and Behavior   57

CHAPTER 5

Interviewing Techniques 83

CHAPTER 6

Adapting Communication to a Patient's Ability to Understand 108

CHAPTER 7

Patient Education 132

CHAPTER 8

Cultural Sensitivity in Healthcare Communication 148

PART III:

Administrative Communication Skills   177

CHAPTER 9

Electronic Communication   179

CHAPTER 10

Fundamental Writing Skills   197

Part I

PRINCIPLES OF COMMUNICATION

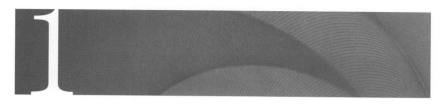

THE COMMUNICATION PROCESS

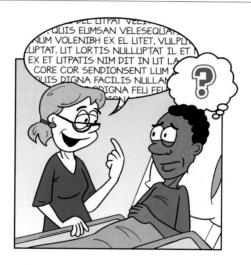

OBJECTIVES

- Explain the importance of effective communication
- Describe the elements of the communication process
- Describe the obstacles to successful communication

If you are reading this book, you are probably an allied health student, and you might be asking yourself the following question: Why should I study communication as part of allied health?

The answer is that as an allied healthcare professional in the 21st century you need to have stronger communication skills than ever before. The standard of care demanded at all points of patient contact requires that you effectively communicate with patients and other members of the healthcare team. This means that you have the skills necessary to ensure clear and compassionate understanding when you encounter a patient in the waiting room, the examination room, on the telephone, or through email. You should also know how to work efficiently and productively as a member of the healthcare team to ensure the highest level of effectiveness in serving patients' needs.

You will be working and living in a society that is more diverse—and more complex—than any society the world has ever known. Serving patients from such a diverse population requires that you have the skills to bridge gaps in communication that earlier generations of allied health professionals could not or did not have to cross.

As an allied health professional in the 21st century, you must not only possess the clinical skills necessary to providing excellent patient care, but you must also master the communication skills essential to ensuring positive health outcomes for patients. At the most basic level, this means that when you encounter a patient, or colleague, that person's message gets to you clearly, and, in turn, your response gets back to that person clearly.

This may sound very simple, but as this book will demonstrate, getting the message clearly from one person to another can involve many sophisticated skills and the ability to overcome obstacles. These are the skills and abilities you will need as a future healthcare professional (HCP).

Therapeutic Communication

For our purposes, *therapeutic communication*, which is the primary focus of this book, *is communication between the HCP and the patient (as well as the patient's family) that takes place to advance the patient's well-being and care*. Therapeutic communication has three main purposes:

1 To collect healthcare–related information about the patient;
2 To provide feedback in the form of healthcare–related information, education, and training; and
3 To assess the patient's behavior and, when appropriate, to modify that behavior.

At any time when you communicate with a patient or their family members, you are engaging in therapeutic communication. As an HCP, you should remain mindful that effective therapeutic communication is always characterized by support, clarity, and empathy.

Any of the following could happen on any day in the doctor's office, hospital, or healthcare center where you will be working:

■ *You greet a new patient and, after escorting them to the examination room, prepare them for the physician who will arrive shortly to give them a physical examination.*
■ *An elderly, hearing-impaired patient comes to your lab needing a pulmonary function test.*
■ *A young mother with an at-risk pregnancy comes in to see you for her biweekly sonogram.*

- *A pharmacist leaves a phone message for the renewal of a patient's prescription.*
- *You have just drawn blood for routine screening from a 4-year-old boy who sits on his mother's lap and screams, "I want my blood back!"*
- *A physician in your practice asks you to contact the radiology department of a nearby hospital to make an appointment for a patient who needs a chest x-ray.*
- *A new patient who has heard great things about one of the doctors in your practice wants an appointment with that doctor, who is not currently accepting new patients.*
- *You answer the telephone and the person on the other end says they are a patient in your practice and that they are currently having chest pains.*
- *A paramedic brings in the unconscious victim of a gunshot wound.*
- *Twenty minutes after a patient on your ward has crashed and been rushed to the intensive care unit, a family member who knows nothing of what has just happened shows up for visiting hours.*

For each of these scenarios to be resolved successfully, effective communication needs to take place.

Effective communication is necessary for any human interaction to succeed. As a healthcare professional, you will need effective communication skills to provide care to patients, and to fulfill your obligations to your supervisor and your co-workers.

A Definition of Communication

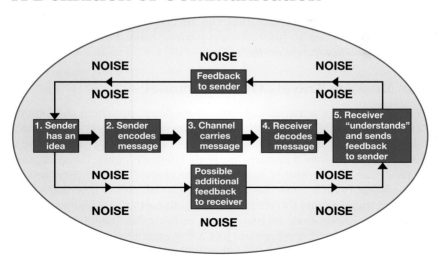

FIGURE 1-1. **The Communication Process.** This figure illustrates the five steps in the communication process and noise, the primary obstacle to the effectiveness of the process.

We can say that *communication is the successful transfer of a message and meaning from one person or group to another.* "Meaning" is of greatest importance in this definition. For this transfer to be successful, both parties in the communication process—that is, the sender of the message and the message's receiver—must agree on the meaning of what is being communicated. This process usually contains five steps. In each of these steps, an effective communicator will take into account possible physical limitations or cultural differences that may inhibit or disrupt communication.

The Five Steps of the Communication Process

The Sender has an Idea to Communicate

This idea to be communicated can be the result of thought or feeling and can be influenced by the circumstances of the current situation, as well as the sender's mood, physical condition, culture, heritage, or background. The sender simply has something they want to communicate to someone else. (For example, *a radiology technologist must instruct a patient on how to place their injured arm on the x-ray table.*)

The Sender Encodes the Idea in a Message

To encode the idea means to put the idea into some form that can be communicated. The sender puts the idea into spoken or written words, or perhaps into hand gestures, body movements, or facial expressions. A good communicator always understands the importance of using words, symbols, or gestures that the receiver will understand. (*The radiology technologist instructs the patient with* words *on how the injured arm should rest on the table.*)

The Message Travels Over a Channel

There is always a particular means, or medium, by which the sender sends the message. This is the *channel*. The sender can choose to use a telephone, speak face-to-face, write on paper or electronic tablet, send a fax or an email, draw a picture, use body language, make facial expressions, or use hand gestures. Sometimes the channel can be disrupted by *noise*. Noise (which is discussed in greater detail later in this chapter) is anything that disrupts the channel's ability to carry the message clearly. Static on a phone line, an improperly printing fax machine, and bad grammar in an email message are just a few examples of channel noise. The effective communicator, however, will always try to minimize noise and ensure that conditions are optimal to send the message by the medium they have chosen. Healthcare professionals must accommodate patients who have impairments in sight or hearing. They must also be able to accommodate those who cannot use the technology on which many channels of communication rely today. (*In addition to words, the radiology technologist uses gestures to demonstrate the arm's proper placement.*)

The Receiver Decodes the Message

The receiver must then make some sense of the message. To do this, the receiver must *decode* the message, that is, translate the original message from its encoded form into a form that the receiver understands. This step in the communication process can be complicated by many factors, all of which are also types of *noise*. For instance, there may be cultural differences between the sender and the receiver. Perhaps the receiver does not have the education necessary to understand the content of the message. Finally, the receiver may have poor listening—and, therefore, poor communication—skills.

There might be physical conditions that prevent the receiver from decoding the message. These can sometimes be actual noises, such as the noise from a nearby construction site or a car horn, a telephone ringing or a baby crying, or even a family member interrupting the patient interview. Other physical conditions that can cause the receiver difficulties include physical sensations, such as an overheated room or a room that is too cold, or any discomfort from pain.

Finally, anxiety or fear can prevent the receiver from being able to concentrate on the message the sender is trying to transmit, again causing a breakdown in the communication process. (*Despite the pain of the injury, the patient tries their best to listen to the radiology technologist's instructions.*)

The Receiver Understands the Message and Sends Feedback to the Sender

The receiver understands the message and provides the sender with feedback, something that says, *I have received your message and I understand it.* This can be verbal or nonverbal—that is, the receiver can say something or make some gesture with their body or hands.

The sender of the original message can enhance this step in two ways. First, they can try to communicate at a time and under circumstances that are convenient to the receiver. Second, the sender can verify that the message has been received and understood, essentially asking of the receiver, *Do you understand me?* An effective communicator should always remain careful not to provide more information than the receiver can process at any one time.

The receiver can also enhance this step by paraphrasing back to the sender the original message, saying, *This is what I think you said.*

(Placing their arm across the table, the patient says to the radiology technologist, "Is this how you want me to do it?")

Finally, the receiver can do nothing, that is, make no response—which is also a response of sorts—in effect telling the sender of the message that they have not received or understood the message. The sender must try again.

Noise

Anything that inhibits effective communication can be labeled *noise*. Although the term can at times refer to actual sound, noise does not have to literally prevent one or both parties from audibly hearing the other. Noise can come in many different forms. For instance:

- The receiver of the message may have some sort of physical pain or discomfort that prevents them from effectively "listening."
- The receiver may be distracted by fear or anxiety about themselves or a family member or friend and cannot effectively concentrate on the message.
- There may be a language barrier or cultural differences that prevent the receiver from understanding the message.
- The receiver may not be interested in what the sender of the message has to say, either through a simple lack of interest or because of other concerns that have a higher priority for the receiver.
- The receiver of the message may be hearing or sight impaired.
- Finally, the channel by which the sender transmits the message may be faulty or may even break down as, for instance, when a phone connection has fuzzy static or when a fax machine runs out of toner.

Ultimately, anything that disrupts the communication process is noise.

An Illustration of the Five-Step Communication Process

The process can be illustrated with one of the examples from the beginning of this chapter. Suppose a pharmacist has called the medical practice where you work and left a voicemail message indicating that a patient wants a refill on a prescription for an asthma medicine that has expired. You transcribe the message and pass it on to the physician. The physician then writes the prescription and places it in the patient's chart. The chart is returned to you so that you can follow up by faxing the prescription to the pharmacy so that the prescription can be refilled.

This one scenario actually contains the communication process in a couple of layers. Let's look at just one layer of this process.

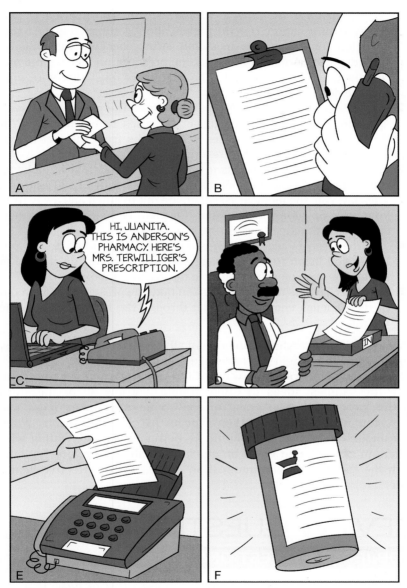

FIGURE 1-2. The Communication Process. (A) *The sender has an idea to communicate*—the pharmacist (the sender) has a prescription that needs to be refilled for one of his customers; **(B)** *The sender encodes the idea in a message*—the pharmacist uses a specialized language to describe the prescription; **(C)** *The message travels across a channel*—the pharmacist uses a telephone and leaves a message on the medical assistant's voicemail at the doctor's office; **(D)** *The receiver decodes the message*—the medical assistant transcribes the voice message into a written message for the doctor (the receiver); **(E)** *Feedback travels to the sender*—the medical assistant takes the approved prescription and sends it by fax to the pharmacist; **(F)** *Success!*

1 *The Sender has an Idea to Communicate:* The pharmacist has received information from the patient about getting a refill on a prescription for an asthma medicine. After checking the patient's records, the pharmacist sees that the prescription has expired and that the doctor must renew it. The pharmacist must, therefore, contact the doctor's office.

2 *The Sender Encodes the Idea in a Message:* The pharmacist uses a specialized language—a language that uses technical terms for drugs and dosage amounts as well as units from the metric system—to describe what the prescription is.

3 *The Message Travels Across a Channel:* The pharmacist picks up the telephone to call the doctor's office. Because it's 12:30 p.m. on a Tuesday, you, the medical assistant, are out to lunch and away from your desk. Speaking on the phone, the pharmacist leaves you a message on the practice's answering system.

4 *The Receiver Decodes the Message:* Having returned from your lunch, you listen to the message and write it down on a piece of paper. You then place the paper in the doctor's inbox.

5 *Feedback Travels to the Sender:* You take the prescription form out of the patient's chart and send it through the fax machine to the pharmacy.

Thanks to the successful completion of all five steps in this communication process, the patient will have an easier time breathing.

We may not always be aware of it, but even when we communicate the simplest ideas to other people, we use all of the steps in this process. A firm grasp of the communication process will help you understand all other aspects of communication. When you understand these, you should be better at communicating with others in general, and you'll be much more able to provide patients with the therapeutic communication necessary for effective health care.

REVIEW QUESTIONS

OBJECTIVE QUESTIONS

1 A patient's deafness can be a form of noise. (*True or false?*)

2 When a nurse asks a patient a question, the patient simply stares back blankly. This is not a form of feedback. (*True or false?*)

3 Sign language is not a channel for communication. (*True or false?*)

4 When a doctor tries to examine a patient with abdominal pain, they ask the patient to rate the pain on a scale of 1 to 10, with 10 being the worst pain imaginable. The patient screams and says, "It's a 10!" That scream is an example of noise. (*True or false?*)

5 In order to encode a message, the sender must have a computer or fax machine. (*True or false?*)
6 A nurse's pager that goes off, displaying a phone number, is not a channel for communication. (*True or false?*)

SHORT ANSWER QUESTIONS

1 Define the word *encode* and provide two examples of its use.
2 List three possible forms of noise that might impair communication in a hospital emergency department waiting room.
3 List three channels a doctor might use to communicate with a patient.
4 Suggest three ways in which cultural differences can inhibit the communication process.
5 Suggest two ways a healthcare professional can enhance communication when explaining to a patient a complicated regimen for taking a medication.

CLINICAL APPLICATION

Alberto Mendez, a 46-year-old man with a family history of heart disease, has shown up 30 minutes late for a routine physical examination. Mr. Mendez does not speak English, but he has brought his 15-year-old daughter with him to serve as an interpreter. After his arrival in the office and before his being shown into the examination room, the front desk receptionist explains to you that he is late because his car was rear-ended by another car as he sat at a red light in a nearby intersection. As a result, the receptionist tells you, Mr. Mendez is very upset. He's now in the examination room waiting for you to interview and prep him for his visit with his physician. When you walk into the examination room to interview him, you sense immediately that he is upset. He sits on the examination table, shaking a fist in the air and speaking heatedly in Spanish with his daughter, who has tears running down her cheeks. Your responsibilities as the medical assistant are to take Mr. Mendez's vital signs—his pulse, temperature, blood pressure, and respiratory rate—and find out if there is anything he wants you to report to the doctor before they come in to examine Mr. Mendez.

1 Identify two steps from the communication process that may take place during this encounter.
2 Based on the information available in the scenario, discuss the factors that may act as noise and impair the communication process.

Fundamental Writing Skills

The final chapter of this book (Chapter 10) provides a thorough review of grammar, a basic overview of effective paragraph construction, and a brief introduction to SOAP (Subjective-Objective-Assessment-Plan) note taking. You can work through the chapter over the course of the semester one section at a time, completing one of the nine sections along with each of the first nine chapters of the book. This step-by-step method will make completing the grammar section easier and less burdensome. At the conclusion of each exercise, you can check your comprehension in the accompanying online answer key.

You will find at the end of each of the first nine chapters a section number for one part of Chapter 10. The section number indicates the section and exercises you are to complete along with the chapter you have just read.

Section 10-1 in the writing skills chapter is the section you should complete at the end of Chapter 1. You can find this section on pages 197–204.

SUGGESTED FURTHER READING

1. Abou-Auda HS. Communication Skills. Retrieved April 25, 2010 from http://faculty.ksu.edu.sa/hisham/Documents/PHCL455/Communication_Skills_Hisham.pdf.
2. Adams C, Jones P. *Interpersonal Communication Skills for Health Professionals*. New York: McGraw-Hill; 2000.
3. Guffey ME. *Essentials of Business Communication*. 7th ed. New York: Thomson; 2006.
4. Losee R. Communication defined as complementary informative processes. *Journal of Information, Communication, and Library Sci*. 1999;5(3):1–15.
5. Ramutkowski B, Booth K, Pugh D, et al. *Medical Assisting: Administrative and Clinical Competencies*. 2nd ed. New York: McGraw-Hill; 2005.
6. Shannon C, Weaver W. *The Mathematical Theory of Communication*. Urbana: University of Illinois Press; 1949.

2

NONVERBAL COMMUNICATION

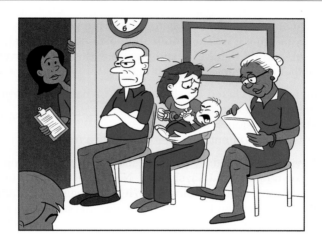

OBJECTIVES

- Describe why the understanding of nonverbal communication is important in health care
- Explain how each of the following may convey nonverbal messages to the observer: gestures, facial expressions, gaze patterns, personal space, position, posture, and touch
- Explain why verbal messages and nonverbal messages must be congruent
- Describe the methods by which the healthcare professional can confirm their interpretation of a patient's nonverbal behavior
- List the proper nonverbal communication skills for the healthcare professional

Communication between healthcare professionals (HCPs) and their patients begins well before they actually say anything to each other. It occurs when the HCP observes the body language of the patient and even when the patient observes the body language of the HCP. Nonverbal communication, which may be unintentional, includes body movements, gestures, and facial expressions. These behaviors convey information that words alone often do not. Have you ever tried to have a sensitive or emotional conversation on the phone or via email? The possibility for misunderstanding is much greater than when you are speaking with someone face-to-face. Why? We rely on nonverbal behaviors to give further meaning to the message. In fact, it is generally accepted that 70% of communication is nonverbal, 23% involves the tone of voice, and only 7% of communication occurs by the chosen words. Nonverbal communication provides a clue to a person's inner thoughts and feelings, and this form of communication is particularly important in stressful situations, as a message of need is most likely to be sent nonverbally.

Imagine entering a waiting room and observing the patients. There are universal, natural behaviors and positions that may convey significant meaning. For example, a patient may:

- Have their arms relaxed on the armrest or have their arms folded tightly across their chest;
- Sit up straight or slouch in a chair;
- Have a pleasant, content expression or have a frown.

Other behaviors exhibited by patients may also be revealing such as nail-biting, toe-tapping, and leg-shaking. No interaction may take place; however, these observations allow the HCP to begin formulating opinions about their patient and the patient's emotional state. As a result, the HCP can adapt their behavior and select responses with which to interact with the patient according to these impressions. For example, the nonverbal behaviors displayed by a seriously ill patient may convey a buildup of feelings, especially fear, anxiety, confusion, or anger. This patient may benefit from extra attention in the form of interest, concern, consideration, and emotional support. The HCP could invite the patient to release their pent-up feelings by talking about their concerns. Therefore, it is essential that the HCP observe and correctly interpret nonverbal behaviors displayed by their patients so that any unspoken messages are not lost.

It is important to remember that one cannot always be sure what certain behaviors indicate. For example, consider the patient who is sitting with their arms folded across their chest. An initial interpretation may be that the patient is angry or impatient. However, one must be mindful that this position could have other meanings. Does it provide them with some form of comfort or the feeling of protection from nearby people? Are they self-conscious about their appearance? Or are they simply cold? Many aspects of nonverbal communication, especially eye contact, are culturally informed and need to be interpreted according to the sender's cultural background. Specific aspects of nonverbal communication related to cultural differences are addressed in Chapter 8, "Cultural Sensitivity in Healthcare Communication."

ROLE **PLAY** **The Waiting Room**

In small groups where two students are the HCPs and other students are the patients, act out the following scenario with regard to the observation of nonverbal behaviors.

Two medical assistants look out into the waiting room of the doctor's office where several patients are waiting. In private, they discuss the following:

- The patient with whom they would most like to interact and why (discuss the nonverbal behaviors conveyed by the patient that made that person appear the most pleasant);
- The patient with whom they would least like to interact and why (discuss the nonverbal behaviors conveyed by the patient that made that person appear the most unpleasant);
- Which behaviors displayed by the patients appeared neutral (discuss the nonverbal behaviors conveyed by the patient that did not send any particular message);
- Which behaviors convey meaning regarding the patient's emotional state?

Nonverbal messages can enhance or interfere with the verbal messages that are delivered. There must be congruency, or consistency, between the verbal and nonverbal messages. If there is conflict, then the nonverbal messages tend to be believed. It is also important to remember that the patient is reading the nonverbal messages transmitted by the HCP. Therefore, the most effective HCPs are those whose nonverbal messages are congruent with their verbal messages. As a result, patient satisfaction with care, patient compliance and health outcomes are improved. In fact, studies indicate that many types of HCPs, including nurses, physical therapists, resident physicians, surgeons, and oncologists benefit from the inclusion of formal instruction in nonverbal communication in their training.

Types of Nonverbal Communication

There are several distinct categories of nonverbal communication, including:

- Kinesics (involving body movement in communication)—gestures, facial expressions, and gaze patterns;
- Proxemics (involving the physical distance between people when they communicate)—territoriality and personal space, position, and posture;
- Touch.

Interestingly, nonverbal messages tend to appear in groups or clusters. For example, a patient's gestures, facial expressions, and posture may all work together to convey the same message.

Gestures

FIGURE 2-1. **Gestures.** Gestures include movements of the head, hands, eyes, and other body parts.

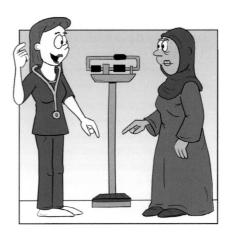

Gestures include movements of the head, hands, eyes, and other body parts. Often used in place of words, gestures are one of the most obvious and common forms of nonverbal communication. For example, a hand extended outward may signify "stop" or "wait" and a finger across the lips may signify "quiet." Gestures may be used when speech is ineffective (e.g., a language barrier) or insufficient (e.g., complex content in the message). Patients who are intubated and mechanically ventilated, are most likely to use head nods, mouthed words, and gestures as their primary methods of communication. Gestures may also be used to relieve stress (e.g., running one's hand through one's hair). Finally, gestures are used to regulate the flow of conversation. For example, a head nod may signify "go ahead" or "continue" and a frown or raised eyebrow may signify confusion. Greater patient–HCP rapport has been reported when the HCP nods their head.

Illustrators are intentional gestures closely associated with speech. They serve to emphasize, clarify, or add to the verbal content of a message as well as to hold the attention of the listener. Illustrators are generally made by movements of the hand. Furthermore, they may serve many different purposes. For example, they may be used to:

- Demonstrate how to hold one's arm during a mammogram;
- Illustrate how to position oneself for an x-ray;
- Indicate where an incision will be located;
- Instruct a patient about how many pills to take;
- Encourage a patient to relax during blood pressure measurement, phlebotomy, or a painful procedure.

Other illustrators may demonstrate how a patient should take a deep breath during spirometry (a method of measuring lung function) or how a patient should open their mouth and say, "Ahhhh."

Gestures may also be involuntary or subconscious. This is referred to as "leakage," when the true feelings or attitudes are revealed by an individual. For example, an 18-year-old football player may say that he is not afraid of the injection or the clinical procedure, but he wrings his hands or shakes his leg.

Many gestures have common interpretations. "Positive" gestures may include thumbs up, winks, handshakes, and fist bumps. These are signs of acceptance, encouragement, appreciation, and friendliness. "Negative" gestures may include looking at one's watch, rolling one's eyes, and tapping one's foot. These are signs of boredom and impatience. The use of gestures is one of the most culture-specific forms of nonverbal communication. In other words, a specific gesture may have very different meanings in different cultures. A gesture interpreted as positive by one individual may be interpreted as negative by another. Care must be taken not to unintentionally offend a patient. These concepts will be discussed further in Chapter 8.

ROLE **PLAY** **Gestures**

With a partner, where one is the HCP and the other is the patient, act out several types of gestures that intentionally or unintentionally convey a message. Discuss the possible interpretations of these gestures. If these gestures were made by a patient, how would you, as the HCP, react? Discuss how these messages may affect how you interact with the patient. If these gestures were made by the HCP, how would you, as the patient, react? Discuss how these messages may affect how you interact with the HCP.

Facial Expressions

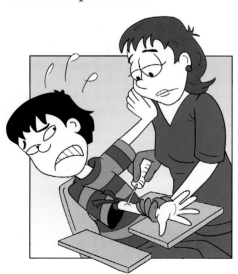

FIGURE 2-2. **Facial Expressions.** Facial expressions provide a rich source of information regarding emotions. Many facial expressions are biologically determined, universal, and learned similarly across cultures.

The human face provides a complex but rich source of information regarding emotions for HCPs as well as patients. These expressions may also be used to punctuate a message or to regulate the flow of conversation between two individuals. Because patients are sometimes reluctant to express themselves verbally, it is essential that HCPs understand and accurately interpret their patient's facial expressions.

The facial expressions of many emotions, such as happiness, sadness, and fear, are biologically determined, universal, and learned similarly across cultures. Consider the small infant that smiles and giggles when happy and frowns and cries when startled, wet, or hungry. These responses are innate, not learned.

Facial expressions are one of the most important and observed nonverbal communicators. The eyes may reflect feelings of joy and happiness or sorrow and grief. A smile conveys a positive attitude and positive feelings. Interestingly, false smiles do not involve the cheeks or the eyes. Various movements of the cheeks, mouth, nose, and brow may express happiness, interest, surprise, fear, anger, disgust, or sadness.

Listeners use facial expressions to provide the speaker with feedback. Facial expressions can show the speaker not only that the listener is interested, surprised, or disgusted by what they have heard, but that they have understood. The speaker is able to monitor these reactions and adapt communication accordingly. During a conversation with a patient, a smile serves as a reinforcer and encourages the patient to continue.

As with subconscious gestures, some people find it difficult to control their facial expressions. The face may "leak" information about a person's true feelings. For example, it may be difficult to hide shock when treating a patient with a horrific wound or to disguise disgust when caring for an incontinent patient. HCPs must learn to control their facial expressions carefully to prevent conveying these potentially hurtful feelings to their patient.

The facial expression of pain is of particular importance to the HCP. Grimaces of pain are not observed in a patient until that patient's threshold of pain is reached. (This threshold level varies among individuals.) The literature suggests that, unfortunately, HCPs have a tendency to underestimate pain when performing clinical assessments. Furthermore, it appears that the more clinical experience one has, the more likely that one will underestimate the level of pain. Interestingly, studies also indicate that people who live with patients who have chronic illness made better assessments of pain than people who had not had that experience. In addition, a patient's voluntary exaggeration of pain in the presence of others may not be meant to be disingenuous, but rather may be a message to elicit care. These findings highlight the importance of the accurate interpretation by HCPs of nonverbal behaviors in their patients who may be in pain.

Facial Expressions

With a partner, where one is the HCP and the other is the patient, act out several types of facial expressions that intentionally or unintentionally convey a message. Discuss the possible interpretations of these facial expressions. If these facial expressions were made by a patient, how would you, as the HCP, react? Discuss how these messages may affect how you interact with the patient. If these facial expressions were made by the HCP, how would you, as the patient, react? Discuss how these messages may affect how you interact with the HCP.

Gaze Patterns

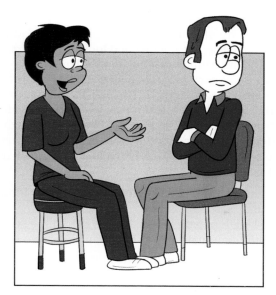

FIGURE 2-3. Gaze Patterns. Gaze may be used to assess how others appear, to regulate conversation, or to express feelings and emotion.

Gaze is a form of communication as well as a method for collecting information. Specifically, it serves three primary functions:

- Monitoring—Assessing how others appear (e.g., a nurse gazing at a very sick patient for clues about their condition), or how a listener is responding to the speaker (e.g., interest, understanding, boredom, confusion)
- Regulating—Using gaze to regulate the conversation such as indicating when it is the other person's turn to speak (When a person finishes

speaking, they tend to look at the listener and the listener perceives this as a cue that it is their turn to speak.)

■ Expressing—Feelings and emotion

Few forms of communication carry more weight than looking a patient straight in the eyes. Eye contact illustrates that the HCP is interested in giving and receiving messages and acknowledges the patient's worth. A lack of eye contact or looking away while the patient is talking may be interpreted as avoidance or disinterest in the patient. On the other hand, staring is dehumanizing and may be interpreted as an invasion of privacy. It may come across as discourteous and even hostile, especially when a patient's appearance has been negatively affected (e.g., when a patient presents with any kind of disfigurement or dermatologic condition). The ability to examine the patient without staring at them and making them feel uncomfortable or self-conscious is a mark of professionalism in a healthcare worker.

Gaze patterns are affected by changes in mood. Sad or depressed people tend to make less eye contact and look down. Gaze also tends to be averted in patients with mental health problems.

There is a strong correlation between looking and liking. Patients who receive longer gazes from HCPs tend to talk more freely about health concerns, present more health problems, and provide more information about psychosocial issues. These findings highlight the importance of considering gaze and its functions during the patient interview.

Normal gaze patterns between individuals in conversation may be characterized as follows:

■ Direct eye contact in a normal conversation occurs for about 50% to 60% of the time.

■ The average length of gaze is usually less than three seconds and the average length of mutual gazes is less than about two seconds.

Therefore, the HCP should look directly at their patient, but not 100% of the time. Strive to establish an amount of eye contact where both you and the patient are comfortable.

■ Speakers spend about 40% of their time gazing at the listener and listeners spend about 75% of their time looking at the speaker with each gaze averaging about eight seconds.

Gaze patterns in listeners last longer because of their function as a social reinforcer and a way to indicate attention.

■ The speaker's gaze is more intermittent with the amount of eye-gazing becoming decreased as the complexity of the topic increases.

This is a potentially important consideration when counseling patients or explaining complex procedures to them.

■ Females tend to look more at the other person than males do.

Gestures, Facial Expressions, and Gaze Patterns

In groups of three to four—one patient, one HCP, and one to two observers—act out each of the following scenarios.

1 A 16-year-old girl goes to a clinic for a pregnancy test, which is positive.
2 A 78-year-old woman has fallen and needs an x-ray of her arm.
3 A 35-year-old Spanish-speaking man arrives at the pharmacy to pick up his medication where he is instructed to take one tablet two times per day.
4 A 40-year-old Vietnamese-speaking woman goes to the emergency room with intense pain in the right side of her abdomen.
5 An 87-year-old man who was the victim of a stroke is paralyzed on the right side of his body and cannot speak. It is 10 a.m. and he is upset because his wife who visits him each day at 9 a.m. has not yet arrived.

Following each scenario, discuss the nonverbal behaviors of the patient and of the HCP. What gestures, facial expressions, and gaze patterns were used to convey messages between the individuals? How did the gestures, facial expressions, and gaze patterns affect the behavior of the patient? How did the gestures, facial expressions, and gaze patterns affect the behavior of the HCP? What was effective in facilitating communication? What impaired communication?

Personal Space

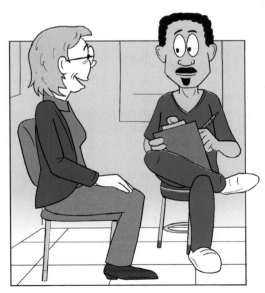

FIGURE 2-4. Personal Space and Position. "Personal distance," or about an arm's length, between the medical assistant and the patient in this illustration is commonly used in healthcare settings. An eye-level position enables the HCP to maintain eye contact with their patient.

Everyone has a personal space, or territory, that provides that individual with a sense of identity, security, and control. People often feel threatened or uncomfortable when that space has been invaded. It may create anxiety or feelings of loss of control. In a healthcare setting, patients are often required to give up this personal space so that they may be properly examined and treated. They may encounter any number of healthcare providers during their time in such a setting, including doctors, nurses, phlebotomists, x-ray technologists, medical imaging specialists, medical assistants, physician assistants, physical therapy assistants, occupational therapists, and nutritionists. Patients who are hospitalized, or who are residents in nursing homes, often share rooms with strangers. These conditions and intrusions may cause a patient who is already sick, weak, or worried to become more anxious or tense.

Approaches that will help to lessen the anxiety created by intrusions and the loss of space include the following:

■ Treat the patient respectfully—Recognize the patient's territory, their belongings, and their right to privacy.
■ Allow the patient to exercise as much control over their surroundings as possible—Allow them to determine whether the lights are on or off, whether the shades are up or down, and whether the door is open or closed.
■ Recognize the patient's need for privacy—Be discrete both verbally and physically. In other words, keep your conversation as private as possible and avoid leaving the patient exposed.

There are four generally accepted distance zones to be considered when interacting with others:

■ Intimate distance = up to 1.5 feet apart. This distance allows the individuals to touch each other. Clinicians often need to enter this zone to examine and care for the patient. HCPs are members of one of the few professions where it is not only legitimate, but necessary, to enter this zone.
■ Personal distance = 1.5 to 4 feet apart (about an arm's length). This is the distance at which personal conversations with soft or moderate voices may take place. The personal distance is commonly used in healthcare settings where a clinical procedure is being explained or a patient is discussing a personal matter.
■ Social distance = 4 to 12 feet apart. This distance is common in business or social settings. Many HCPs may maintain a social distance during a consultation.
■ Public distance = more than 12 feet apart. Used in larger events, this distance is intended to separate the speaker from the listener.

Clearly, the far side of the social distance and the public distance are inappropriate when dealing directly with patients and discussing their health issues. Both intimacy and privacy may be lost at these distances. There are no set rules for HCPs to follow in every situation with a patient. However, the HCP should be sensitive to the distance norms for different situations and allow the patient to participate in establishing these distances whenever possible. When a patient feels that their space has been inappropriately invaded, they may use a shift in body position or use eye contact to send the message.

Allied health professionals may perform many personally invasive tasks during the course of their interaction with patients, such as taking vital signs, giving injections, withdrawing blood, or performing an ultrasound. The HCP will find it helpful to explain any procedure that requires entering the patient's personal space before beginning the procedure. In this way, it is less threatening to the patient, it gives the patient a sense of control and dignity, and it builds a sense of trust in the HCP.

Position

Another important factor to consider when speaking with a patient is position. There are several best practices that will facilitate and enhance the communication process. It is helpful to maintain a close but comfortable position, perhaps about an arm's length from the patient. For example, in an examination room or triage area, have the patient sit in a chair while you sit on a stool that can move across the floor. In this way, you will maintain access to any materials and forms necessary for the visit, you will maintain eye-level conversation, and you will help the patient feel listened to and cared for. Conversely, standing over a patient may convey a message of superiority. Too much distance between the HCP and the patient may be interpreted as avoidance. Finally, moving away from the patient may be interpreted as dislike, disinterest, boredom, indifference, or impatience.

Most interactions between the HCP and the patient require face-to-face communication. This direct orientation increases patient satisfaction and understanding, especially when the patient is anxious. Conversely, an indirect orientation (facing away from the patient) may be perceived as dominance by the patient and could make them feel less comfortable and be less forthcoming.

A position leaning slightly toward the patient expresses warmth, caring, interest, acceptance, and trust. In fact, HCPs who lean forward have been rated as having higher rapport with their patients. The opposite is true for HCPs who lean backward.

Personal Space and Position

In groups of three to four—one patient, one HCP, and one to two observers—act out each of the following scenarios.

1 A medical assistant greets a patient, brings them into the examination room, and asks a few initial questions as to the reason for their visit to the doctor.
2 A patient is hospitalized with a severe form of gastroenteritis and shares a room with three other patients. An RN asks the patient pointed questions about their vomiting and diarrhea.

In terms of personal space and body position, discuss the nonverbal behaviors displayed by the patient and the HCP. What behaviors displayed by the HCP were effective in facilitating communication with the patient? How did these behaviors make the patient feel? What behaviors impaired communication with the patient? How did these behaviors make the patient feel?

Posture

FIGURE 2-5. **Posture.** Posture refers to the position of the body and limbs as well as muscular tone. Posture may reveal a great deal about emotional status.

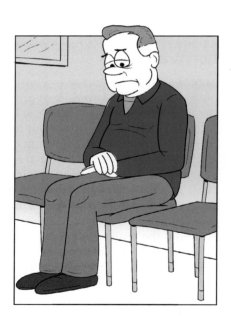

Posture refers to the position of the body and limbs as well as muscular tone. The posture of a patient may reveal a great deal about their emotional status. For example, depression or discouragement is characterized by a drooping head, sagging shoulders, low muscle tone, and the appearance of sadness or fatigue. Conversely, anxiety may be characterized by increased muscle tone where the body is held in a rigid and upright manner. Patients tend to tighten up in fearful or unknown situations. Interest is conveyed by leaning forward with the legs drawn back, while boredom may be conveyed with a lowered head, outstretched legs, and a backward-leaning position. Finally, avoidance and rejection are displayed by a *closed body posture*. In this case, the patient crosses their arms and legs, leans back as if to create distance, and may even turn their body away from the HCP.

It is important that the HCP appear confident as this will enhance the trust that the patient has in them. A crucial aspect for showing confidence is the maintenance of a relaxed and *open body posture*. This posture is also perceived as more friendly, warm, and inviting. In fact, HCPs have been rated as having a greater rapport with their patients when their arms are uncrossed and symmetrical (i.e., arms loosely at their sides when standing or resting on the arms of their chair or in their lap when sitting) and their legs uncrossed. When sitting, the HCP should face the patient and lean slightly forward.

 Posture

With a partner—one patient and one HCP—take turns playing the patient and, using only nonverbal communication, act out each of the following: anger, fear, disgust, happiness, sadness, and surprise. Correctly interpret the displayed emotion. Discuss how, as an HCP, you would react to these messages. Discuss how, as the patient, these messages conveyed by the HCP made you feel.

Touch

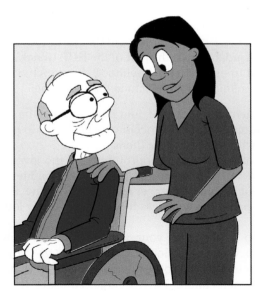

FIGURE 2-6. Touch. Touch is critical in establishing rapport between the HCP and their patient.

Caring for patients often involves some form of touch. Most obviously, it serves as a critical tool for examining (e.g., medical assistant taking blood pressure), diagnosing (e.g., radiography technologist positioning a patient for an x-ray or a phlebotomist withdrawing blood), treating (e.g., physical therapist assistant manipulating a patient's limb or a nurse applying a dressing on a wound), or simply caring for (e.g., CNA helping a patient to eat or to dress) the patient. Touch also has many other important functions in health care as it may serve to:

- Ease a patient's sense of isolation;
- Decrease patient anxiety;
- Demonstrate caring, empathy, and sincerity;
- Offer reassurance, warmth, or comfort;
- Enhance the rapport between the HCP and the patient;
- Supplement verbal communication.

Clearly, touch is critical in establishing rapport between the HCP and the patient. Interestingly, surveys have shown that many patients want to shake their physician's hand when they first meet. However, it is also important to remember that touch may evoke negative reactions in some patients. Not everyone likes to be touched, as it may make them feel embarrassed, uncomfortable, or threatened. Cultural differences are important factors in determining a patient's receptivity to touch and will be considered in Chapter 8.

There are no set rules for determining when to touch or not to touch patients. Furthermore, there is no universally accepted meaning that may be derived from a given touch. Interpretation and receptivity to touch will depend on several factors, and the use of touch will require the exercise of good judgment on the part of the HCP. General guidelines that can be followed to enhance the likelihood that touch will be perceived positively in the clinical setting include the following:

- Tell your patient when, where, and how they will be touched during an examination or clinical procedure. This helps to put your patient at ease and will avoid startling them.
- Use a form of touch that is appropriate for the given situation. For example, placing your hand on the arm or shoulder to ease a distressed patient or family member may be comforting. However, touching an angry patient may be less helpful than simply letting them vent their feelings.
- Use touch to supplement your verbal message. However, do not replace words with touch alone. That may lead the patient to feel that the importance of their problem is diminished or that you are being superficial or demeaning. For example, consider the case where a patient describes the amount of pain felt in their neck following a car accident. If the HCP were to simply pat the patient on the back, the

patient may interpret this gesture as placating and not really caring. Conversely, the same touch accompanied by the words "Let's prescribe some medication for that pain" would be interpreted quite favorably.

■ Do not use a touch gesture that implies more intimacy with a patient than is desired. When a gesture suggests a degree of intimacy that is not shared, it will likely result in discomfort. When touching a patient of the opposite gender, it is advisable to have a colleague or a family member of the patient in the room in order to prevent any misunderstanding.

■ Observe and assess the recipient's response to the touch. Negative responses may include pulling away, a startled look or frightened appearance, a tense facial expression, or other anxious gestures or behaviors. You may safely assume that a patient has a positive response to touch if they appear to relax or seem more comfortable.

■ The person who touches may be perceived as having enhanced status. Therefore, it is important that the HCP remain mindful of its possible effect on the power dynamic between them and the patient. In some instances, the patient may feel a reduced sense of independence or autonomy.

 Position, Distance, and Touch

With a partner—one patient and one HCP—act out the following scenario.

A 45-year-old man is in a deep sleep in his hospital room. It is 2 a.m. and he needs to be given his medications.

Discuss the way in which the HCP used position, distance, and touch during the interaction. As the patient, which practices were received favorably? Why? Which practices were received unfavorably? Why?

Proper Interpretation of Nonverbal Communication: Congruency with Verbal Messages

Successful communication requires congruency between the verbal and nonverbal messages. In other words, the two messages must be in agreement, or consistent, with each other. For example, if a patient says, "Okay," while shaking their head, then they are sending mixed messages. If the patient says, "Yes, I understand," while maintaining a confused facial expression, then once again, they are sending mixed messages. As indicated previously, the nonverbal message is usually accepted as the intended message. If the patient is made aware of the conflict, then they may be encouraged to revise their response. In this way, the HCP may better appreciate what the patient is feeling:

■ "You say that you are fine, but your frown tells me something else."
■ "I notice that you are smiling. Can you tell me how you really feel about this diagnosis?"

The message of a patient's nonverbal behavior is lost unless it is observed and interpreted correctly. The HCP should remain mindful that the misinterpretation of a patient's nonverbal behavior can lead to more misunderstanding than simply ignoring it. When interacting with a patient and the meaning of their nonverbal behavior is unclear, the HCP must make this observation known. Consider the patient who is sitting with their arms folded across their chest and is turned away (Refer to Figure 2-3.). The HCP may take one of several approaches:

■ Make a nonjudgmental observation of their behavior—"You have folded your arms across your chest." or "You are not looking at me."
■ Ask for clarification—"What does this mean for you?" or "Can you tell me what you are feeling?" or "What's going on?"
■ Offer an explanation or interpretation of the patient's nonverbal behavior—"Are you angry or upset?" or "I can see that you are perhaps frightened or anxious."

In some instances, behavioral observation may be the only mechanism by which the HCP may derive information from a patient. For example, a patient may be speech impaired (e.g., due to stroke or intubation), too young (e.g., in the case of an infant), too sick (e.g., due to a semi-conscious or delirious condition), or simply unwilling to communicate verbally.

Proper Nonverbal Communication Skills for the Healthcare Professional

In order to create the best environment for effective communication with your patient, you must be mindful of your own nonverbal messages that may be conveyed to the patient. The most obvious nonverbal message conveyed by the HCP involves their appearance. Ideally, your body should be clean, your clothing should be clean and neat, and your breath and body should have a pleasant or benign odor. Heavy perfumes, aftershaves, piercings, and tattoos are inappropriate in the clinical setting.

Another nonverbal message that may be conveyed by the HCP involves facial expressions. Few of us realize how we look in random or unguarded moments. For example, try to recall a photograph of yourself that was taken when you were unaware and were not posing or smiling. Did the captured expression accurately convey your feelings at the time? Personal concerns and worries or work stress may be unintentionally apparent on our faces and in how we interact with our patients. In other words, an HCP who is actually quite warm and friendly may at times appear abrupt and unapproachable and not even be aware of it. The HCP should be cognizant of these possibilities and attempt to maintain friendly or neutral facial expressions when interacting with their patients.

For a summary of the factors that contribute to the development of an ideal environment for communication between the HCP and their patients, see Table 2-1.

TABLE 2-1

Factors that Contribute to the Development of an Ideal Environment for Communication between the HCP and Their Patients

- Wear professional attire and maintain good hygiene.
- Offer the patient a firm handshake and a warm greeting.
- Sit down when speaking with the patient.
- Ensure privacy when speaking with the patient.
- Assume a position of about one arm's length from the patient.
- Maintain a posture that is relaxed but attentive. When seated, lean slightly forward and be still but not motionless. Keep your hands visible.
- Eliminate barriers between you and the patient.
- Maintain a demeanor that is warm and friendly.
- Maintain an attitude of confidence and professionalism.
- Maintain eye contact with the patient. This will confirm your willingness to listen and will acknowledge the patient's worth.
- Encourage the patient with affirmative head nods as opposed to listening without expression. This not only prompts the patient to continue and provide more information, it makes the patient feel understood and empathized with.
- Recognize the different forms of nonverbal communication that may be conveyed by the patient. In many cases, there are similarities in the way that most people physically react and express themselves. However, the HCP must remain mindful that various gestures, facial expressions, or postures may have many different meanings. Avoid making assumptions and try to confirm the proper interpretation of a patient's nonverbal behaviors.
- Observe the patient's reactions toward you. This will provide feedback about your own nonverbal behaviors.

REVIEW QUESTIONS

OBJECTIVE QUESTIONS

1 Another term for nonverbal communication is _____ .
2 Most forms of nonverbal communication are cross-cultural and are interpreted similarly between people of different ethnic backgrounds. *(True or false?)*
3 As much as 70% of communication is in the form of nonverbal communication, which is particularly important in stressful situations such as illness or medical emergencies. *(True or false?)*
4 When verbal messages and nonverbal messages are not congruent, the verbal message tends to be believed. *(True or false?)*
5 Two types of nonverbal communication that help to regulate the flow of conversation include _____ and _____ .
6 In order to put the patient at ease, it is important that the HCP maintain direct eye contact with the patient during the entire course of the conversation. *(True or false?)*
7 When discussing a sensitive topic or describing a clinical procedure, it is appropriate for the HCP to maintain a _____ distance between themselves and the patient.
8 The HCP who leans slightly forward during the conversation has a better rapport with their patients. *(True of false?)*

SHORT ANSWER QUESTIONS

1 Describe some instances in which the use of gestures facilitates the communication between the HCP and their patient.
2 Discuss the characteristics of "good eye contact" between the HCP and their patient.
3 What approaches help to ease the anxiety in a patient created by intrusions and the loss of personal space when hospitalized?
4 A hospitalized patient is in the radiology department for a computed tomography (CT) scan. The radiology technologist must position the patient in the machine. Discuss the best practices that should be employed by the HCP. What practices should be avoided?
5 A 6-year-old boy has fallen off his bicycle and sustained a deep cut on his arm that requires stitches. Discuss how the HCP should approach this patient to clean and treat the wound. Include appropriate forms of touch between the HCP and the boy. What other nonverbal behaviors will enhance the interaction and communication between the HCP and the boy?
6 Why is it essential to properly interpret the nonverbal communication displayed by a patient?

CLINICAL APPLICATIONS

1 Watch an episode of your favorite medical drama on television with the sound turned off. Describe how the HCP interacts with different types of patients. Describe the emotions of the HCP and the patient in terms of each of the forms of nonverbal communication. Describe how the HCP interacts with other HCPs. How do these interactions differ from those occurring with the patients?

2 A 28-year-old professional baseball player tells you that he is not worried about having arthroscopic surgery on his knee. Describe any nonverbal behaviors that would be inconsistent with this verbal message. How will these observations cause you to adapt your approach with this patient?

3 A phlebotomist must draw blood from a 3-year-old child. Discuss the nonverbal behaviors that may be employed to help put the child at ease. Discuss the behaviors that may be employed to help put the child's mother at ease.

4 Recall your most recent experience in a healthcare setting, either as a patient or as the HCP. If you were the patient in this experience, describe the nonverbal behaviors exhibited by the HCP. How did these behaviors make you feel? Is there anything that the HCP may have had done differently? If you were the HCP in this experience, describe the nonverbal behaviors exhibited by a specific patient. How did the patient's behaviors lead you to adapt your behaviors in order to promote your communication and rapport with the patient?

Fundamental Writing Skills

The section in the writing skills chapter you should complete at the end of Chapter 2 is Section 10-2. You can find this section on pages 204–208.

SUGGESTED FURTHER READING

1. Abou-Auda HS. Communication Skills. Retrieved April 2010 from http://faculty.ksu.edu.sa/hisham/Documents/PHCL455/Communication_Skills_Hisham.pdf.
2. Adams CH, Jones PD. *Interpersonal Communication Skills for Health Professionals.* 2nd ed. New York: Glencoe McGraw-Hill; 2000.
3. Ambady N, Koo J, Rosenthal R, et al. Physical therapists' nonverbal communication predicts geriatric patients' health outcomes. *Psychol Aging.* 2002; 17(3):443–452.

4. Beck RS, Daughtridge R, Sloane PD. Physician-patient communication in the primary care office: A systematic review. *J Am Board Fam Pract.* 2002; 15:25–38.

5. Berger B, Diggs AM. Immediacy—part 2, nonverbal communication. *U.S. Pharmacist.* 2008; 25:8–12.

6. Everitt, K. Good Patient Communication May Prevent Medical Errors, 2007. Retrieved April 2010 from http://www.sfc-acs.org/information/GoodPatient-CommunicationMayPreventMedicalErrors.doc.

7. Freeman R. Communicating effectively: some practical suggestions. *Br Dent J.* 1999; 187(5).

8. Frew MA. *Comprehensive Medical Assisting: Competencies for Administrative and Clinical Practice.* 3rd ed. Philadelphia: F. A. Davis Co.; 1995.

9. Green MS. Intention and authenticity in the facial expression of pain. *Behav Brain Sci.* 2002; 25:460–461.

10. Griffith CH, Wilson JF, Langer S, et al. House staff nonverbal communication skills and standardized patient satisfaction. *J Gen Intern Med.* 2003; 18(3): 170–174.

11. Happ MB, Tuite P, Dobbin K, et al. Communication ability, method, and content among nonspeaking nonsurviving patients treated with mechanical ventilation in the intensive care unit, *Am J Crit Care.* 2004; 13(3):210–220.

12. Indiana University (2006, January 30). You Don't Say: Patient-doctor Nonverbal Communication Says A Lot. *ScienceDaily.* Retrieved April 2010 from http://www.sciencedaily.com/releases/2006/01/060130155029.htm.

13. Journal of the American Medical Association and Archives Journals (2007, June 12). Survey: Most Patients Want to Shake Hands With Their Physicians. *ScienceDaily.* Retrieved April 2010 from http://www.sciencedaily.com/releases/2007/06/070611164246.htm.

14. Keir L, Wise BA, Krebs C. *Medical Assisting, Administrative and Clinical Competencies.* 5th ed. Clifton Park, NY: Thomson Delmar Learning; 2003.

15. Lindh WQ, Pooler MS, Tamparo CD, et al. *Comprehensive Medical Assisting, Administrative and Clinical Competencies.* 4th ed. Clifton Park, NY: Thomson Delmar Learning; 2009.

16. Lussier MT, Richard C. Doctor-patient communication, the medical interview. *Can Fam Physician.*, 2004; Retrieved April 2010 from http://www.cfpc.ca/cfp/2004/Jan/vol50-jan-clinical-4.asp.

17. Milliken ME, Honeycutt A. *Understanding Human Behavior, A Guide for Health Care Providers.* 7th ed. Clifton Park, NY: Thomson Delmar Learning; 2004.

18. Nishizawa Y, Saito M, Ogura N, et al. The non-verbal communication skills of nursing students: Analysis of interpersonal behavior using videotaped recordings in a 5-minute interaction with a simulated patient. *Jpn J Nurs Sci.* 2006; 3(1):15–22.

19. Cegala DJ, McGee DS, McNeilis KS. Components of patients' and doctors' perceptions of communication competence during a primary care medical interview. *Health Commun.* 1996; 8(1):1–27.

20. Northouse LL, Northouse PG. *Health Communication, Strategies for Health Professionals.* 3rd^d ed. Stamford, CT: Pearson Education; 1998.

21. Preston P. Nonverbal communication: do you really say what you mean? *J Healthc Manag.* 2005; 50(2).

22. Smithco H. Actions speak, the power of non-verbal communication. *TherapyTimes*, Retrieved April 2010 from http://www.therapytimes.com/content= 5201J64E48BEB6841.

23. Solomon P. Congruence between health professionals' and patients' pain ratings: a review of the literature. *Scand J Caring Sci.* 2001; 15(2):174–180.

24. Stewart M, Brown JB, Hammerton J, et al. Improving communication between doctors and breast cancer patients. *Ann Fam Med.* 2007; 5(5): 387–394.

25. Tamparo CD, Lindh WQ. *Therapeutic Communications for Health Care.* 3rd ed. Clifton Park, NY: Thomson Delmar Learning; 2008.

26. Williams D. *Communication Skills in Practice, A Practical Guide for Health Professionals.* Bristol, PA: Jessica Kingsley Publishers; 1997.

3

VERBAL COMMUNICATION

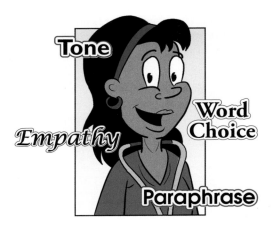

OBJECTIVES

- Explain the purposes of using clear language for effective verbal communication with patients
- Identify practices for effective verbal communication with patients and other healthcare providers
- Develop skills for listening and paraphrasing
- Explain why providing empathy and understanding to the patient is so important
- Demonstrate the methods of questioning the patient

The lack of effective communication is the single most common cause of patient complaints. As a healthcare professional (HCP), you simply must have good verbal communication skills. Being able to communicate effectively with patients and colleagues can make all the difference between a career that succeeds and one that does not succeed. From the initial job interview through the promotion process, a professional's ability to communicate verbally is continually assessed by hiring committees and supervisors. Most important, though, is that an HCP who has strong communication skills will always be more effective in helping patients. However, it is important to remember that being a good verbal communicator is not simply a matter of having a large vocabulary or the ability to use highly technical language. Being a good communicator consists of maximizing the effectiveness with which you understand what others are trying to tell you and accurately conveying what you want to say. As a future HCP, you cannot afford to have weak verbal communication skills.

Definition of Verbal Communication

Verbal communication is the use of spoken words and sounds to successfully transfer a message from the sender to the receiver.

The Purposes of Using Clear Language for Effective Verbal Communication with Patients

Content and Word Choice

The content provides the meaning of what a speaker intends to convey to the listener. For effective communication to take place, the content must be as clear as possible, and this means that the speaker must first of all have a clear understanding of what they mean to say. When the speaker does not have a clear sense of what they intend to say, the

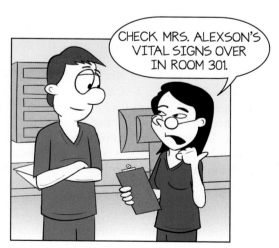

FIGURE 3-1. The Directive Tone. Authoritative and judgmental, the directive tone is used to give orders, exert leadership, and pass judgment.

receiver of the information can become confused. Consider the following example:

Imagine for a moment that you are a patient who has come in to have blood drawn for a fasting cholesterol. It is 8:30 on Monday morning and you have not eaten since before 9:00 on Sunday evening. You are hungry and irritable. You have been shown into the room where you will have the blood drawn, and the young female phlebotomist whom you expect to draw the blood simply stands there in front of you, hands on hips, looking a bit puzzled. After a moment, you get the sense that she does not really know why you are there. She obviously has not bothered to read your chart before the encounter. She stands there looking at you and says, "I don't know. What are we going to do today? Take a urine? A throat culture? Some blood? Let's see." Your confusion, even anger, would be justified. You could very well wonder whether this HCP was even competent to perform the service you have come in for.

In addition to knowing what they intend to say, the speaker must use words that accurately reflect their intended message. The speaker should avoid unclear, ambiguous, or unnecessarily technical language.

Let's suppose that the phlebotomist mentioned above has read your chart and the doctor's orders. She knows you have come in for a fasting cholesterol. She sits you down in the phlebotomy chair and says, "Don't you dare move! I'm going to stab you in the arm with one of my big old needles and take some of that blood." Again, your confusion and anger would be justified. Even if the phlebotomist said something like, "I need to make this withdrawal for an HDL, LDL, triglyceride, as well as a total cholesterol," your frustration would be understandable.

An HCP who can communicate effectively will have a clear sense of what they want to say, and they will say it using the appropriate word choice.

"I'm going to draw some blood for a fasting cholesterol. Please place your arm across the padded bench so that your palm is up. Now make a fist with your hand. I'll tell you when you can open it. There will be a small pricking feeling at first and then it will be over."

This explanation indicates the professionalism of the HCP when interacting with the patient. The patient will respond more positively to this than they will to flippant or overly technical explanations.

Grammar and Pronunciation

The speaker should speak in grammatically correct sentences. Incorrect grammar can impede the clarity of the message and, just as important, can diminish the confidence the listener has that the speaker knows what they are talking about. The same holds true for pronunciation. Each setting in which human interaction takes place has agreed-upon pronunciations for words commonly used, and it is important that the speaker remain mindful of the setting and use appropriate pronunciation. In a healthcare setting, standard English pronunciation is appropriate. Correct pronunciation enhances understanding and rapport between the speaker and listener. Incorrect pronunciation inhibits understanding and can cause mistrust.

Tone

The tone with which the HCP speaks to the patient is vital to the therapeutic relationship because it indicates an understanding of the patient's needs and enhances the HCP's ability to meet those needs. Tone accomplishes this by helping both parties to understand their relationship and its tenor. Generally speaking, the tone the HCP uses should be relaxed and conversational, helping to establish rapport with the patient. Beyond that, there are three types of tone worth exploring: Expressive, Directive, and Problem-Solving.

Expressive Tone

An expressive tone is spontaneous, emotional, and uninhibited. We use this tone, for instance, when we express our feelings, tell jokes, or complain—when we socialize. When having coffee or dinner with friends, or when confiding in a family member, we talk about what we like or do not like, what we want or do not want. We express ourselves, and we use the expressive tone.

For example, while sitting in a café with a friend we might say something like, *"I really wish I had studied harder in math so I could do my own taxes."*

or,

"Can you believe how goofy Professor Martin's haircut looks?"

or,

"I hate my boss. He never tells me I've done a good job, even when I work all night on projects. He can only say something about my work when he doesn't like it."

This is generally not a tone of voice the HCP should use when speaking to patients. First, for reasons explained more fully below, using the expressive tone is often inappropriate in a healthcare setting because it takes the focus of the discussion off the patient and puts it on the HCP. The HCP should make every effort to let the patient know that the patient's needs are the reason for the visit. Second, research indicates that patients do not usually appreciate an emotional or even joking tone from their HCPs. Relaxed and conversational, yes; full of feeling and funniness, no. The patient has come in for a serious reason, and they want the interaction with the HCP to be direct, empathic, and professional.

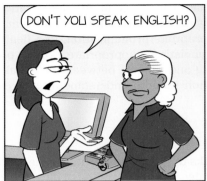 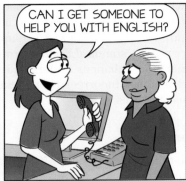

FIGURE 3-2. The Directive Tone versus The Problem-Solving Tone. (A) Using the directive tone with a patient can cause misunderstanding; **(B)** The problem-solving tone builds rapport, showing the patient you are there to help.

Directive Tone

A directive tone is authoritative and judgmental. This is the tone one uses to give orders, exert leadership, or pass judgment. When a supervisor at work asks you to complete a task, explains the scheduling needs for the coming month, or clarifies areas on your annual performance review in which you could improve, they use the directive tone. The directive tone is an indication that there exists a difference in professional rank between the speaker and the listener.

For example, a nursing supervisor in a hospital's internal medicine clinic may say to a medical assistant, *"Mr. Jimenez [a patient] is in Examination Room 3 and needs his vitals taken. Please take care of that right away."*

or,

"Can you see to it that Ms. Higgins is taken down to radiology at 2:00? They're expecting her for a head CT."

or,

"Mark [another medical assistant] needs to take Saturday off for a family funeral. Can you come in to work Urgent Care from 8:00 to 5:00?"

The directive tone is generally not an appropriate tone for the HCP to use when speaking to patients. Patients come into the practice seeking expert treatment that includes understanding and empathy on the part of the healthcare team. As part of that treatment, patients frequently need to receive instruction from their HCPs. However, it is important for the HCP not to confuse providing patient instruction with giving the patient orders. Consider the following two examples involving a nurse whose patient has an upper respiratory infection. The patient's doctor has prescribed an antibiotic to fight the infection. In the first example, the nurse orders the patient to comply, and in the second, the nurse instructs the patient about the benefits of compliance.

Ordering the patient: *"I'm telling you. Don't miss a single dose of this pill. If you do, your infection won't go away and you'll feel even worse."*

Explaining to the patient: *"Taking these pills regularly will achieve the best results. You'll do a better job of fighting the infection."*

The patient is much more likely to respond positively to what the nurse says in the second example and is, therefore, much more likely to comply with the instruction.

| ROLE |
| **PLAY** |

Hand Washing

With a partner, where one is an HCP and the other a patient on an in-patient infectious disease ward at a large hospital, act out the following scenario in which the HCP must instruct the patient in proper hand washing. Using their hands, the HCP must show the patient how to wash, and then instruct the patient while they wash their hands. Take turns using the Directive tone and a Tone that explains to the patient the benefits of good hand washing. Discuss which is more effective and why.

Problem-Solving Tone

A problem-solving tone is rational, objective, and unbiased. This is the tone we use to indicate to the listener that we are using the analytical portion of our brains to come to the correct answer about a certain set of circumstances. When we provide complicated street directions to a friend who is visiting from out of town, describe a missed homework assignment to a classmate who was absent, or explain how to download a computer file, we use the problem-solving tone. This is the tone the HCP uses most frequently when serving patients' needs. A significant part of the allied health professional's job consists of verbally collecting important information from the patient and providing explanations and solutions to the patient. The problem-solving tone is what the patient rightfully expects from the HCP.

Consider the following pairs of examples and choose the statement or question in each that would be more effective for an HCP to use with a patient. One statement or question in each pair uses the problem-solving tone, and one uses another tone, either the expressive or the directive.

Statement A: *"Eating so many cheeseburgers every day for the past five years could be a contributing factor in your high blood pressure. Cheeseburgers contain a lot of sodium, and sodium is often associated with high blood pressure."*

Statement B: *"Eating so many cheeseburgers is going to make you fat and give you a heart attack. Is that what you want?"*

In the first set of examples, Statement A uses the problem-solving tone and is more effective, whereas Statement B, which uses the expressive tone, is likely to offend the patient.

Question A: *"Don't you speak English?"*
Question B: *"Can I get someone to help you with English?"*

In the second set of examples, Question A uses the directive tone and is less effective. The patient is likely to feel more comfortable responding to Question B, which uses a problem-solving tone, than to Question A, which uses a directive tone that sounds almost accusatory. In each case the patient would be more receptive to what the HCP is saying when a problem-solving tone is used to convey or retrieve information.

ROLE
PLAY

Using the Correct Tone

With a partner, use your best problem-solving tone to play the role of the HCP and counsel the patient about one of the following situations. Try to avoid using either the expressive or directive tone.

- **The HCP is a dental hygienist who has to explain to the patient the benefits of daily flossing.**
- **The patient has poison ivy and wants to scratch the welts. The patient should not do this under any circumstances.**
- **The patient should not try to clean their ears with sharp metal tweezers because doing so can cause serious injury.**

Emphasis

By this time, it should be clear that how you say something is often just important as what you want to say. Even within a sentence, the emphasis you place on certain words or parts of a sentence can lead to vastly different interpretations by the patient. Consider the following versions of the same sentence: *I believe you will get better*. Each sentence has a different word emphasized.

- *I* believe you will get better.
  - The emphasis here suggests that the speaker is perhaps alone in believing the patient will get better.
- I *believe* you will get better.
  - This sentence has an emphasis that says the speaker may have some doubt about the patient's improvement, but really wants to believe it.
- I believe you will get *better*.
  - This last version's emphasis on the word "better" suggests that the speaker may not actually doubt the words they are saying about the patient's improvement, but that the speaker still wants to cheer the patient on.

Clearly, in each of these cases *how* the speaker says what they want to say is as important as *what* they want to say.

Small Talk

This is a good place in our discussion to mention *small talk*. Small talk is what we say to each other before we begin to discuss the business at hand. Hence the expression, *"Let's cut the small talk and get down to business."* Small talk is talk about the weather, the local sports team, why the subway train was delayed and the patient was late getting to the doctor's office. Small talk is not talk about emotional, personal, or controversial subjects. An HCP can use small talk to help a nervous patient feel more at ease, taking some of the feelings of pressure off the patient. When the patient is more comfortable, they will be better able to discuss their case. If, for example, a family member is present in the examination room during the visit, the HCP can engage them in small talk to build rapport with the patient. One should always keep in mind, though, that small talk should be limited as it is not the purpose of the patient's visit. Small talk should be viewed and used as a tool for building rapport with the patient.

Using Commentary

There will inevitably occur brief periods during the visit when the HCP must focus on some task that is part of the care process but is not part of directly engaging the patient in questions and answers. These tasks can range from the unpleasant, such as changing a colostomy bag or cleaning an infected intravenous (IV) site, to the mundane such as preparing an x-ray machine or entering data into the patient's file on a computer. Such moments of "downtime" can become awkward for the patient if they pass in utter silence. It is, therefore, helpful to the process if the HCP briefly comments on what they are doing, just to keep the interaction alive and allow the patient to remain engaged in the active role they take in their own care. Such commenting, moreover, can ease fear and reduce anxiety for the patient.

One should always remember, though, that strategies such as small talk and commentary are best used to build and strengthen rapport with patients. When used too frequently or for excessive amounts of time, these techniques can become distracting to the patient.

Important Practices for Effective Verbal Communication with Patients and Other HCPs

Send a Clear Message

An effective message is a clear message. Patients come to see their HCP for the most serious of reasons—their health—and the information

FIGURE 3-3. Actively Listening to What the Patient Says. Actively listening and confirming for the patient that you have understood them is crucial to establishing rapport and showing empathy.

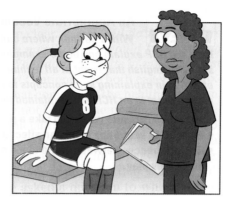

Developing Skills for Listening and Paraphrasing What the Patient Says

Perhaps the most important part of good listening is paraphrasing. To paraphrase is to use your own words to repeat what someone else has said. Good paraphrasing skills are essential to effective communication. An HCP should use paraphrasing for several important reasons.

A Test of the Message for the HCP

Paraphrasing back to the patient what the patient has said provides the HCP with an opportunity to verify that they have understood what the patient has said. By paraphrasing, the HCP is allowing the patient to either confirm that the HCP has the correct information or point out inconsistencies or gaps in the information. Under optimal circumstances, this is simply to verify that the HCP has received the same message that the patient has intended to send. However, circumstances are not always optimal. A patient may be angry, confused, in pain, speech impaired, or in some other condition that makes it more difficult for them to get their message across to the HCP. It is important that the HCP try to understand exactly what the patient is trying to communicate. Consider the following example, in which a 16-year-old female high school student shows up in an orthopedist's examination room complaining of knee pain.

The orthopedic nurse is with the girl evaluating her before the doctor arrives. The girl's mother is also there.

The girl is clearly distressed. The nurse can see that she has been crying. The girl's mother, who wears an angry expression on her face, sits stonily silent in a chair nearby.

"I just have to make varsity soccer this year," the girl tells the nurse, her speech rushed. "I'll just die if I don't. I'll disappoint everybody." Her glance lands on her mother for a second. "But I can't even do a push pass, let alone any kind of kick," she continues. "Every time I lift my leg to push the ball with the inside of my foot my right knee pops and turns to the right. It hurts so much I just fall down." She looks again at her mother and asks her, "You didn't have these problems when you were playing, did you?"

This is a complicated and messy situation, but the nurse should remember first of all why this patient has come in: with a complaint of knee pain. The nurse needs to focus directly on that when paraphrasing the girl's words, but the nurse should be mindful that not to acknowledge the anguish she is feeling at the prospect of failing to make the team will damage the communication process. The girl is telling the nurse she is upset, but still, the girl is there because of the pain in her knee.

A Test of the Message for the Patient

The patient listens to their HCP's paraphrase, checking to see that the paraphrase is what the patient intended to say and that the HCP understands. As in the preceding example of the soccer player, what the patient wants to say and what comes out are not always identical. The orthopedic nurse needs to focus on what they believe the patient wants to say. The girl wants to hear the nurse respond to the problem of her knee pain, despite the fact that most of her energy is taken up with talking about her fear of not making the team. The nurse in this example could show effective communication skills by responding as follows:

"We'll do everything we can to help you feel better so you can make the team. I can tell how important that is to you. But I want to make sure I understand exactly what happens when you move your leg or put pressure on your knee in certain ways. Now, you say that in lifting your leg to push the ball with your instep you put pressure on your knee, and then your knee makes a popping sound and turns outward to the right. And it hurts?"

Hearing this response, the girl can verify that what she wants to tell the nurse is what the nurse is actually hearing.

A Building of Rapport—a Human Connection

Paraphrasing what the patient says helps to build trust between the patient and the HCP. The HCP shows engagement with the patient's case, validating the patient's concerns. The patient understands from this interaction that the HCP is focused on the patient and cares about them. The patient is then more likely to slow down and listen carefully to the HCP. The young girl in our example hears in the voice of the nurse empathy and concern. The girl can tell that the nurse is not going to judge her in any way about making the soccer team or about anything else. The nurse is there to help the girl with the pain in her knee. The girl can correctly infer all of this from the clear and appropriately focused paraphrase that comes from the nurse. The girl feels more comfortable with the nurse and is able to tell the nurse in detail about the knee. The girl can let go of the superfluous emotional worry that accompanied her into the room.

"It hurts here," the girl says, pointing to an area just to the inside of the patella. She turns her knee a bit outward. "And it moves out like this. Ouch!"

Focusing on the Patient and Keeping the Patient Talking

Paraphrasing what the patient says reinforces the point that the healthcare encounter is occurring for the purpose of helping the patient. The patient is made to understand that everything they and the HCP say has to do exclusively with the patient. When the patient clearly understands this, they are at greater ease in the therapeutic relationship, becoming better able to play a role in their own care. Patients typically have a lot to say about their own case, even if they do not seem to at first. However, once the HCP has helped the patient to understand that a complete focus on the patient's case is entirely appropriate, the patient will feel more comfortable and open up. The would-be soccer player in our example is able to focus exclusively on working with the nurse to evaluate the knee before the doctor arrives. Their discussion contains none of the fluster and frustration that filled the room when the nurse first came in.

ROLE **PLAY**   **Good Paraphrasing**

With a partner, take on the roles of patient and HCP. Practice paraphrasing one of the following scenarios (the student playing the patient should try to be imaginative):

- In the morning when the patient wakes up, the patient's ears feel clogged and there is a slight pressure inside the head. When having this feeling, the patient cannot hear his or her own words clearly when speaking. The problem does not go away until after breakfast.
- The patient feels nauseous when taking medicine before meals. The problem is not so bad toward the end of the day, but first thing in the morning the feeling is at its worst.

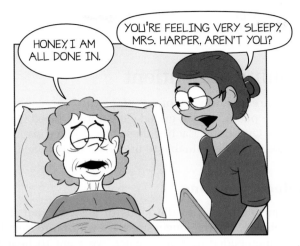

FIGURE 3-4. Good Paraphrasing. Good paraphrasing verifies that you have understood the patient and is essential to building rapport and showing empathy, all of which can lead to a better outcome.

Providing Empathy and Understanding to the Patient

By now, it should be obvious that by *paraphrasing* we do not mean merely mechanically repeating back what the patient says in slightly different words. In paraphrasing, the HCP should also try to convey something of the emotion that is inherent in what the patient said. The HCP achieves this by thinking critically about what the patient actually says and trying to understand. This speaks to the larger issue of showing empathy. To show empathy to the patient is to show that you understand how the patient feels—to the point of being able to put yourself in their place and feel what they feel. The patient will almost always tell you how they are feeling, even when they are trying not to. Either through nonverbal or verbal means, the patient will communicate, which means that the HCP must be an effective listener and observer.

The Differences between Empathy and Sympathy

Empathy is sometimes confused with sympathy, but there are important differences between these two concepts. To feel empathy is to feel what another person is feeling, that is, to be able to put yourself in another's shoes. To feel sympathy is to have an awareness of what another person is feeling, and to feel sadness or pity at that other person's suffering, that is, to feel sorry for that other person. Showing empathy for a patient can build rapport, whereas showing sympathy can show distance between the HCP and the patient, and even cause negative feelings on the patient's part toward the HCP.

Questioning the Patient

The HCP has three main types of questions they can use to elicit information from the patient: Open-ended Questions, Closed Questions, and Multiple Choice Questions. Each of these has its place in effective verbal communication, and it is valuable to understand how each works.

Open-ended Questions

Open-ended questions lead to the kinds of answers that the HCP will want to paraphrase, that is, longer answers with more detail and emotion. We use open-ended questions when we want to hear the whole story. Open-ended questions most frequently begin with the words "how" or "what." Consider the following examples of open-ended questions:

- "What do you say to a patient who is angry about waiting?"
- "How do you feel when you go into a test without having studied?"
- "How do you feel about working with elderly people?"
- "What made you want to go into an allied health profession?"

Open-ended questions encourage the patient to further discuss issues of concern, and these questions can be very helpful in coming to a complete understanding of the patient's needs. There are also times, however, when the HCP wants very specific information from the patient, and at these times the HCP may use closed questions.

Closed Questions

Closed questions prompt a short and focused answer, frequently just a "yes" or a "no," or perhaps a one-word answer. They are especially helpful in filling in gaps in what the patient says, or in keeping track of the patient's information for medical record purposes. Consider the following examples of closed questions:

- "What city do you live in?"
- "Which arm hurts?"
- "Can you hear me?"
- "Does it hurt when I touch that?"

An effective communicator will understand when it is appropriate to use open-ended and closed questions. Frequently, HCPs are working against time constraints. It is, therefore, important that they recognize the point at which they have sufficient information derived from open-ended questions and can conclude the encounter by filling in any gaps with closed questions.

Multiple Choice Questions

Multiple choice questions provide the patient with alternative options from which to choose. These can be helpful in allowing the patient to collaborate with the HCP in the management of their care, thereby helping patients to feel more empowered in making care-related decisions. Multiple choice questions can also be helpful when working with patients who are withdrawn, depressed, or anxious, in that they aid the patients in taking steps in prioritizing their actions. Consider the following example, in which a nurse's aide works with a geriatric patient living in an assisted living facility:

HCP: *"What would you like to do first this morning, Mrs. Martinez? Would you like to eat breakfast, bathe, or watch television?"*

Patient: *"I want to watch television while eating breakfast. There's that new talk show on I want to see. I can take a bath later. I might even take a nap before my bath."*

One possible disadvantage to multiple choice questions is that they can sometimes feel too complicated to the patient, almost as if more than one question were being asked at a time, which can lead to the patient's confusion or frustration. Finally, elderly patients may have trouble with multiple choice questions as they can often grow impatient with questions that seem to delay the next step in their care.

Some Do's and Don'ts of Verbal Communication

Use the Patient's Name

First impressions are important, and using the patient's name in greeting them at the initial meeting is a way to make a good first impression. It shows respect. As an HCP who has effective communication skills, you understand the importance of establishing rapport with the patient. Using the patient's name at the initial meeting and at the beginning of each subsequent meeting is crucial to that rapport. To not use the patient's name is to indicate that just who they are is not very important to you. This is not the impression you want to make.

Do Not Interrupt the Patient

As an HCP you want to receive important information from the patient. When the patient begins to tell you their story, remember to let them finish. Interrupting a speaker indicates that the listener does not think the speaker's message is very important. An HCP who has effective communication skills will allow the patient to finish speaking without unnecessary interruption. To allow the patient to finish speaking is to reinforce the message that you are there to serve the patient's needs.

Do Not Give the Patient Unsought or Unrelated Advice

When a patient arrives for a visit, they have generally come for a specific reason—a reason that has to do with their health and medical care. As a HCP, it is your task to stay focused and speak only to the patient's case as it pertains to this context. You may notice or be aware of any number of issues surrounding the patient's appearance or personal life that have nothing to do with the patient's reason for the visit. It is inappropriate to give advice—no matter how well meaning—on any issue other than that for which the patient has made the visit.

Do Not Talk about Yourself Instead of Talking about the Patient

Remember: It is the patient's case you are there to discuss. You may think you have real insight based on your own personal experience of the issue for which the patient has made the visit. However, it is inappropriate to talk about yourself or your experience in the matter that concerns the patient. The reason for the visit is to serve the patient, not you.

Do Not Tell the Patient You Know How They Feel

Telling the patient you know how they feel is not the same as showing empathy. To show empathy is to show that you understand what the patient is feeling—even to the point of feeling what the patient is feeling—which is a primary means to building rapport. It is important to always remember that you and the patient are there to serve the patient's needs first. To tell the patient you know how they feel is to one-up the patient, diminishing the significance of their feelings.

REVIEW QUESTIONS

OBJECTIVE QUESTIONS

1 Patients complain more about dirty examination rooms than anything else in health care. *(True or false?)*

2 It is always a good idea for the allied health professional to assert authority and use the directive tone when speaking to patients. *(True or false?)*

3 An HCP whose mother had the very same complaint as the patient should tell the patient about their mother because that will help the patient feel more comfortable. *(True or false?)*

4 There are two types of tone in addition to the directive tone; the other two types are the _____ and the
_____ .

5 A closed question will generally prompt a one-word answer. *(True or false?)*

6 To show a patient empathy means to show the patient you understand how they are feeling. *(True or false?)*

7 Using slang is an effective way of connecting with a patient you have never met but who belongs to an ethnic group you think you understand. *(True or false?)*

8 Repeating the expression "Let me tell you what I think you're going through" is a not good way to show empathy to the patient. *(True or false?)*

9 Repeating back to the patient what they have told you wastes valuable clinical time. *(True or false?)*

SHORT ANSWER QUESTIONS

1 Why is the problem-solving tone more effective than the expressive tone when discussing a patient's skin rash?

2 Name two instances when commentary might be useful during a patient encounter.

3 Why is it important to use a patient's name?

4 Discuss the differences between the following statements: (A) "Don't eat that rich ice cream if it always gives you a stomachache"; (B) "The lactose in ice cream and other dairy products may contribute to the stomach pain you often experience."

5 Describe the ways in which paraphrasing can enhance the patient–HCP relationship.

6 Why is it important to not interrupt the patient in the middle of their history?

7 Provide three examples of open-ended questions and explain why each is an open-ended question.

CLINICAL APPLICATIONS

1 A 47-year-old man has morbid obesity, diabetes, and high blood pressure. He seems to understand the regimen of medications the doctors have prescribed for him, and he seems to comply. However, he is having problems controlling his eating. He loves fast food,

especially the triple cheeseburgers with bacon and chocolate milk-shakes from a local restaurant. What would be the appropriate tone to use with this patient? Explain your answer, providing examples.

2 A 35-year-old man, accompanied by his wife, has come for blood draws in the lab where you are a phlebotomist. The man tells you he is terrified of needles. What would be appropriate to say to him? Explain your answer.

3 A 68-year-old woman has arrived for a scheduled abdominal computed tomography (CT) scan in the radiology department where you work as a tech. A part of the process of preparing the patient for the scan is to have her ingest a contrast agent in the form of a drink—sort of a pharmaceutical milkshake. She has had CT scans before and has consumed contrast, but she is convinced that since that last CT she has developed an allergy to the agent. She is terrified of the drink. She has no rational reason for believing she suddenly has an allergy, and she should drink the solution as soon as possible if she is to have her scheduled scan in 30 minutes. What would be the appropriate way to speak to this patient about the prospect of drinking the contrast? Explain your answer.

Fundamental Writing Skills

The section in the writing skills chapter you should complete at the end of Chapter 3 is Section 10-3. You can find this section on pages 208–214.

SUGGESTED FURTHER READING

1. Abou-Auda HS. Communication Skills. Retrieved April 23, 2010 from http://faculty.ksu.edu.sa/hisham/Documents/PHCL455/Communication_Skills_Hisham.pdf.
2. Adams CH, Jones PD. *Interpersonal Communication Skills for Health Professionals*, 2nd ed. New York: Glencoe McGraw-Hill; 2000.
3. Beck RS, Daughtridge R, Sloane PD. Physician-patient communication in the primary care office: a systematic review. *J Am Board Fam Pract.* 2002; 15: 25–38.
4. Buller MK, Buller DB. Physicians' communication style and patient satisfaction. *J Health Social Behav.* 2007;28(4):375–388.
5. Bush K. Do you really listen to patients? *RN.* 2001;64(3):35–37. Retrieved April 23, 2010 from Research Library Core database.
6. Cegala DJ, McGee DS, McNeilis KS. Components of patients' and doctors' perceptions of communication competence during a primary care medical interview. *Health Commun.* 1996;8(1):1–27.

7. Ezell J. How do I deliver hard truths? *Nursing*, 2003;33(7):66. Retrieved April 23, 2010 from Health Module database.
8. Freeman R. Communicating effectively: some practical suggestions. *Brit Dent J.* 1999;187(5).
9. Frew MA. *Comprehensive Medical Assisting: Competencies for Administrative and Clinical Practice.* 3rd ed. Philadelphia: FA Davis Co; 1995.
10. Goldberg MC. If we're lucky, the patient will complain. *Am J Nurs.* 1995; 95(2):52. Retrieved April 23, 2010 from Research Library Core database.
11. Gordon S, Buresh B. Nursing in the right words. *Am J Nurs.* 1995;95(3):20. Retrieved April 23, 2010 from Research Library Core database.
12. Heery K. Straight talk about the patient interview. *Nursing.* 2000;30(6): 66–67. Retrieved April 2010 from Health Module database.
13. Hynes R. Finding the words: when a nurse understands grief. *Am J Nurs.* 2007;107(5):88. Retrieved April 2010 from Research Library Core database.
14. Keir L, Wise BA, Krebs C. *Medical Assisting, Administrative and Clinical Competencies.* 5th ed. Clifton Park, NY: Thomson Delmar Learning; 2003.
15. Lindh WQ, Pooler MS, Tamparo CD, et al. *Comprehensive Medical Assisting, Administrative and Clinical Competencies.* 3rd ed. Clifton Park, NY: Thomson Delmar Learning; 2006.
16. McConnell EA. Sticks and stones...the wrong words can hurt. *Nursing.* 1998; 28(10):HN20–HN21. Retrieved April 2010 from Health Module database.
17. Milliken ME, Honeycutt A. *Understanding Human Behavior: A Guide for Health Care Providers.* 7th ed. Clifton Park, NY: Thomson Delmar Learning; 2004.
18. Northouse LL, Northouse PG. *Health Communication, Strategies for Health Professionals.* 3rd ed. Stamford, CT: Pearson Education; 1998.
19. Patients value friendly nurses. *Aust Nurs J*, 2004;11(11):38. Retrieved April 2010 from Health Module database.
20. Richard P J. Keep it simple: A plea for plain talk. *RN.* 1994;57(10):96. Retrieved April 2010 from Research Library Core database.
21. Seifert PC. Communication—speaking, surfing, and smiling. Association of Operating Room Nurses. *AORN Journal.* 1999;70(4):558–561. Retrieved April 2010 from Health Module database.
22. Skylark-Langton T. Finding the right words. *Nursing.* 2006; 36(10):44–45. Retrieved April 2010 from Health Module database.
23. Solomon P. Congruence between health professionals' and patients' pain ratings: a review of the literature. *Scand J Caring Sci.* 2001;15(2):174–180.
24. Stewart M, Brown JB, Hammerton J, et al. Improving communication between doctors and breast cancer patients. *Ann Fam Med.* 2007;5(5):387–394.
25. Tamparo CD, Lindh WQ. *Therapeutic Communications for Health Care.* 3rd ed. Clifton Park, NY: Thomson Delmar Learning; 2008.
26. Ufema Joy. "Can opener" approach? *Nursing.* 2005;35(11):14–15. Retrieved April 2010 from Health Module database.
27. Williams D. *Communication Skills in Practice, A Practical Guide for Health Professionals.* Bristol, PA: Jessica Kingsley Publishers; 1997.

Part II

CLINICAL COMMUNICATION SKILLS

4

PROFESSIONAL COMMUNICATION AND BEHAVIOR

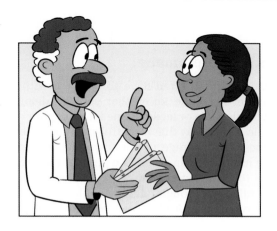

OBJECTIVES

- Identify the benefits of effective professional communication and behavior
- Describe the interpersonal skills that are essential for the successful healthcare professional
- Discuss effective therapeutic communication skills
- Explain roadblocks to therapeutic communication
- Discuss strategies for effectively working with patients who may be angry or anxious
- Describe strategies for effective communication with other members of the healthcare team
- Explain the Health Insurance Portability and Accountability Act (HIPAA) and discuss the privacy issues surrounding HIPAA

A healthcare professional (HCP)—any professional, for that matter—needs to have effective interpersonal skills. These are the skills one relies on most in order to have successful interaction with other people. These skills—which include tactfulness, courtesy, respect, empathy, genuineness, appropriate self-disclosure, and assertiveness—usually do not stand alone but rather exist in concert with one another. What's more, these skills are often considered by many observers to be indicators of a person's character or personality, as they can often reveal just what the sources are of that person's ability to show compassion and caring for others. Most important of all, though, is that in order to become better at communicating in these ways one must often be prepared to grow personally as well as professionally. An allied health professional who exhibits one of these skills as part of effective communication tends to exhibit others as well.

Essential Interpersonal Skills for the Healthcare Professional

Tactfulness and Diplomacy

In the workplace you will often have to disagree with what someone says to you, or let someone know that you are displeased by some action. When you disagree or let someone know of your displeasure, you should always do so in a way that is tactful and diplomatic, that is to say, in a way that does not disparage, or put down, the other person and their actions. We live in a society in which the popular culture seems to value more and more the blunt statement, or even the put-down. Television and movies are filled with tough-talking people, some of whom work in the healthcare professions or play roles of those who do, and who are favorably portrayed for "telling it like it is" or "shooting from the hip," usually getting the last nasty word in. In the real world of work, however, such blunt talk cannot only hurt others' feelings but can also land you in professional trouble. Let's suppose, for example, that you work on an internal medicine unit in a large hospital. At the nurse's station, a colleague of yours has been gossiping to you about the recent break-up of the supervising nurse's marriage. Your colleague has begun to tell you

FIGURE 4-1. Tactfulness and Diplomacy. Idle workplace gossip is inappropriate, and you may need to use tactfulness and diplomacy to remove yourself from such situations.

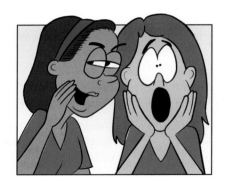

detailed private information—information you really should not know—about your supervisor. You need to remove yourself from this conversation by saying something that is tactful and diplomatic.

You could say to your colleague, *"This is probably something I shouldn't know, and besides, I have to attend to some of my patients. Please excuse me."* By saying this, you would demonstrate tact and diplomacy. You would let the other person know two things: first, that you do not want to engage in idle workplace gossip, and second, that you are there to work and serve the needs of the patients.

Courtesy and Respect

In all of your interactions with colleagues and patients—indeed, in your interactions with all other people—you should show courtesy. In all situations, large and small, you should show consideration for other people's feelings and needs. You show courtesy when you do such things as making room at the table in the nursing station for another nurse who has to sit down to write their notes at shift's end; asking a patient if they need anything while they wait in the examination room a few minutes for the doctor; and offering to get a blanket for the patient who looks a bit cold while sitting in a wheelchair waiting to be taken down to radiology for x-rays. Showing courtesy is an important part of having good workplace manners.

When you show respect for another person, you show that you value that person. When a patient or colleague receives respect from you, they feel that they are important to you. If they are your colleague and they feel you respect them, they will work more effectively with you. If they are your patient and feel your respect, they will be more compliant and more able to help you serve them. You can show respect to others by using both nonverbal and verbal signals. Nonverbally, you can show respect to another person by shaking hands when meeting, and especially by showing that you are paying attention to them: by maintaining a good posture toward them when they speak to you, by facing them, and by making appropriate eye contact with them. Verbally, you can show respect by using an appropriate title, such as Dr., Mr., Ms., or Mrs., and by using their name. You can show respect to another person by giving them your undivided attention when interacting with them.

Empathy

As discussed in Chapter 3, to show empathy is to show that you understand—to the point of feeling—how another person feels. When showing empathy to colleagues and patients, you demonstrate use of all of the important skills discussed so far in this chapter—tactfulness, courtesy, and respect—but you also show that you care. Your empathy tells the other person that you are there to fully acknowledge what they are feeling and that, within the appropriate limits of your power, you will try to provide support and care. You show empathy to colleagues by showing that you carefully listen to what they tell you and that you do your best to understand. You show empathy to patients by showing them that you are paying attention to everything they attempt to communicate to you, and by effectively and completely paraphrasing back to them what they have said.

Genuineness

There is simply no substitute for showing genuineness, or being genuine. To be genuine is to be completely yourself when dealing with others—to be completely open and honest—in all of your words and actions. Friends and loved ones, family members, colleagues, and patients will all know it when you are being genuine with them—and they will know it when you are not. By being genuine, you let others know that they are getting the real you, that you are not putting on any sort of act, or putting up any sort of front. When you are genuine in human interactions, you do not just go through the motions, but you engage fully. Colleagues sense your genuineness when you show that you care about the job you do, and you care about their ability to do theirs. Patients sense your genuineness when you show them courtesy, respect, and empathy, and you show that you are doing your very best to serve them and their needs.

Appropriate Self-Disclosure

To self-disclose is to open up, or show something, about one's self. When you self-disclose to another person, you reveal something about yourself. Generally, we self-disclose when we want to show others that we have experiences similar to theirs, and by doing this we show them that we have something in common with them. We believe this brings us closer to other people. As an HCP, you will have opportunities to self-disclose to colleagues and patients, but you should be thoughtful and cautious about when and how you do this. Self-disclosure is best used when it does two things: first, it shows another person that you have had an experience similar to theirs, thereby illustrating something you have in common with that person; and, second, it has significance because it allows you to show empathy for what that other person is feeling as a result of their experience. In other words, self-disclosure is most effective when you use it almost as a form of paraphrase: you describe to the other person an experience because you recognize that it is parallel to theirs, and you make clear that you are mentioning it only because it is helping you to understand the other person and have empathy for what they are feeling.

For example, a patient who must lose weight for health reasons tells you about the difficulty they have controlling their eating during the winter holidays. At work there are cookies and cakes on every desk and table; after work there are the parties where they and their co-workers eat and drink; and at home there are large family meals with lavish desserts. The patient loves to eat.

You also love to eat and feel the same holiday temptations, and you see in this exchange an opportunity to share this experience with the patient in the service of their health care. In self-disclosing to the patient, you should be careful to avoid the following:

1 Telling a story about yourself simply for the sake of telling a story about yourself;
2 Telling a story that is not about you but about the holiday eating problems of someone else the patient does not know;
3 One-upping the patient by trying to outdo their story on the pitfalls of holiday eating;
4 Removing the focus in any way from the patient.

An appropriate self-disclosure might go like this:

"Every year from mid-November to mid-January I also worry about my eating habits. I have to be careful because everywhere I go

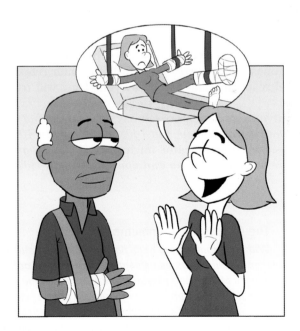

FIGURE 4-2. Appropriate Self-Disclosure. When self-disclosing to the patient, you should be careful not to one-up them with your story.

there seems to be another plate of cookies—and I love cookies. I have to watch out. If I take a cookie whenever I feel like it, I can eat 30 or more in a day, and then I never know how many calories or how much sugar I have taken in. I just can't start—not even one—without it getting out of control. Do you feel that way? I did, and I had to come up with a strategy."

Such a response shows the patient that you have listened carefully to them and that you are showing empathy for the way they feel. Such a response will help the patient feel more comfortable talking about important issues surrounding this part of their health care.

Assertiveness versus Aggressiveness

As an HCP with effective communication skills, you will need to be assertive in your communication style, that is, you will need to be able to comfortably and confidently express your ideas, opinions, and feelings while still respecting the ideas, opinions, and feelings of others. To be an assertive communicator is to be able to stand up for what you believe is right without any undue anxiety about what others may think of you. It is important, however, not to confuse an assertive communication style with an aggressive communication style. When disagreeing with a colleague, an assertive communicator will use clear and direct language while remaining relaxed and respectful, whereas an aggressive communicator can tend to use confrontational and even sarcastic language, while maintaining a tense and often superior attitude. When you use an assertive style, you tell listeners that while you may disagree you remain honest and courteous with them. Their response, in turn, will be to feel respected and valued by you. They will trust you more easily.

An assertive communicator will say, *"I understand what you're saying and your point of view, but I just don't agree with you."*

An aggressive communicator might say, *"I don't agree with you because you're obviously wrong and your opinion is ridiculous."*

ROLE **PLAY** **The Aggressive Communicator**
With a partner, where each has an opposing point of view, choose a subject about which you can disagree, such as stem cell research or the appropriateness of cosmetic plastic surgery to reduce the signs of aging—or your own topic—and practice arguing your point of view from each side of the issue with one of you taking the role of the assertive communicator and the other the aggressive communicator. Switch roles. Can you each remain assertive in the face of aggressive communication?

Effective Therapeutic Communication Skills and Strategies

Just as there are qualities one can possess to be a more effective communicator, there are skills and strategies you can develop to optimize therapeutic communication with the patient. Some of the more important of these are listed here.

Remaining Silent with the Patient

There are times when a patient will need to gather their thoughts or work to formulate what they want to tell you. As an HCP, you will need to develop the important skill of remaining silent while a patient works out what they want to say. The patient has to feel free of pressure while doing this in your presence.

Remaining Nonjudgmental

During a visit a patient may reveal personal attitudes or beliefs with which you do not agree. It is important during such times to remember that your responsibility is to assist the patient in managing their health care. Your responsibility is not to approve or disapprove of the patient's beliefs. For example, a patient who suggests considering such treatment options as alternative medicine, including herbal cures and even folk remedies, deserves the same respectful, empathic, caring, and nonjudgmental treatment as the patient who ascribes to the most conventional treatments of traditional Western medicine.

Showing Acceptance of What the Patient Tells You

While a patient tells you their history and discusses any issues relating to their case, you should make every indication that you are listening carefully. This includes such nonverbal behaviors as body language, facial expression, and eye contact as discussed in Chapter 2, but it also includes small verbal cues you can give the patient when appropriate and without interrupting, such as saying, *"Yes. I understand,"* and *"Please tell me what happened next."*

Giving Recognition

You should always provide the patient with recognition for positive changes and improvements in any area concerning their case. Such positive reinforcement encourages the patient to take a positive attitude toward the management of their health and treatment. A patient who is obese and who has made progress in losing weight will respond positively to the recognition you provide, as will the chronic smoker who gives up cigarettes.

Offering of Yourself

As an HCP, you must always make clear to the patient that your primary responsibility is to serve their healthcare needs, and that your priority is to make yourself professionally available to the patient by providing compassion and empathy.

Giving the Patient the Opening

When working with patients, you will frequently find it necessary to allow the patient an opportunity to initiate discussion of an important topic, or even the reason for the visit. You can do this effectively by asking open-ended questions, such as, "What concerns would you like to talk about?" or "What brings you in for your visit today?"

Leading the Discussion

The patient may stop short of telling you everything you need to know, perhaps out of fear, embarrassment, or any other of the roadblocks discussed in this chapter. In such instances, you must be prepared to lead the discussion with the patient by gentle prods, such as "Please go on," or "Tell me what happened next."

Making Observations

Without appearing to be judgmental, you should be ready to make your perceptions of the patient and their condition known. For example, if a patient presents with a swollen knee but does not tell you the history behind the swelling, you should be ready to say, "Your knee is swollen. What happened?"

If the patient is uneasy or tense about discussing this, asking them about the source of the tension is appropriate.

Encouraging Communication

Always ask the patient to make explicitly clear what they are feeling. Patients frequently assume that because they are sitting on an examination table in front of the HCP that the HCP knows what the patient is feeling. Encourage the patient to make clear just what is going on so that you have a complete picture of their condition. Doing this will also give you the opportunity to provide the patient with empathy and compassion, as well as help you to learn about other as-yet unrevealed issues.

Paraphrasing

As discussed in Chapter 3, always paraphrase back to the patient what they have told you. This will enhance understanding and build rapport.

Roadblocks to Therapeutic Communication Part I—The Healthcare Professional's Behavior

Therapeutic communication—that is, communication that advances the patient's well-being and care—is the primary reason for all interactions between the HCP and the patient, and the HCP must understand that everything they do or say sends a message to the patient. Certain communication behaviors that are appropriate in social settings may not be appropriate in a clinical setting. Such inappropriate behaviors are often called roadblocks to therapeutic communication because instead of helping the communication process as the HCP or patient might hope, they actually impede communication.

Providing Easy Reassurance

When confronted by a patient's unease or distress, an HCP's first impulse as a fellow human being may be to provide reassurance with the intention of soothing the patient's unease. For example, an HCP may want to comfort a patient who is about to hear results on an important test, such as a biopsy to rule out a cancer diagnosis. It is inappropriate to provide easy reassurance by saying something like, *"Don't worry about anything. I know it's all going to turn out just fine."* The HCP should resist this impulse because such an attempt to make the patient feel better may be inappropriate for two reasons. First, the patient has the right to feel any way they may feel and such reassurance diminishes the patient's feelings. Second, the reassurance the HCP wants to provide may give the patient false hope in the face of a negative outcome. A more appropriate response to the patient would be to say, *"You know that whatever the result, you have us here and all of the staff on our healthcare team by your side. We're here to help you every step of the way."*

Providing Empathy and Not Easy Reassurance

In groups of three to four—in which one is a patient, one an HCP, and one or two are observers—act out the following scenario: The patient, who initially presented with chronic headaches, has had a head computed tomography (CT) scan in the past week and is now in the examination room waiting for the doctor. The nurse is preparing the patient for the encounter with the doctor. The patient is ridden with anxiety about what the doctor will say about the CT scan. The nurse naturally wants to show empathy, compassion, and caring without giving easy reassurance. Act out an example of easy reassurance, as well as effective strategies for showing empathy and compassion. Discuss how the patient felt in each case. How was providing empathy more effective than showing easy reassurance?

Minimizing the Patient's Feelings

The HCP should be also careful to avoid saying anything that diminishes or makes light of the way a patient may be feeling. The HCP's job is to listen attentively and show empathy for the patient, thereby opening up the channel to effective therapeutic communication. A patient who feels that the HCP does not take the patient's feelings seriously will not trust the HCP.

Approving/Disapproving

Approving or disapproving of the patient can falsely give the patient the impression that a power relationship exists between them and their

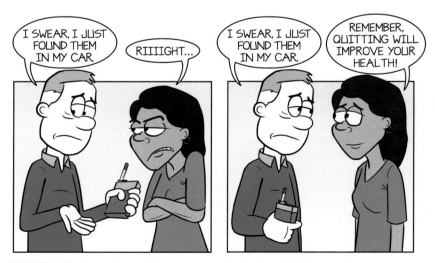

FIGURE 4-3. **Approving or Disapproving of the Patient. (A)** Disapproving can give the false impression that a power relationship exists between the HCP and the patient; **(B)** Explaining the health benefits of certain behaviors helps the patient manage their care.

HCP. An HCP who approves of (as distinct from giving recognition for) a patient's actions can lead the patient to believe that certain behaviors will be rewarded with praise from the HCP. This is inappropriate. Conversely, an HCP who shows disapproval of a patient's actions can cause the patient to feel as if the HCP is passing some sort of moral judgment on the patient. This is also inappropriate. Either of these behaviors can cause the patient to feel as if their relationship to the HCP has to it an aspect of rewards and penalties, and this is entirely inappropriate. The patient's relationship with the HCP exists exclusively to serve the patient and help them manage their healthcare needs.

 The Ex-Smoker

With a partner—one of you is the nurse and the other the patient—play out the following scenarios in which the patient explains that they have either continued to not smoke or relapsed.

Scenario I: The nurse must provide positive reinforcement without seeming to approve of the patient who has gone a whole year without smoking.

Scenario II: Without seeming to disapprove, the nurse must help the patient understand the importance of not smoking after the patient confesses to having relapsed and begun smoking again in private when family members are not around.

What are the most effective behaviors the nurse can show toward the patient? What are others that would be less effective?

Agreeing/Disagreeing

Either agreeing or disagreeing with the ideas, feelings, and thoughts of the patient is an ineffective communication behavior because it turns the discussion of the patient's health into a matter of the patient's being right or wrong. The patient is not coming into the medical practice to meet a kindred spirit who shares their opinion or to argue a point with an antagonist who opposes the patient. The healthcare process should never become about the patient being right or wrong, but should be about helping the patient manage their healthcare needs.

Giving Your Own Advice

You should never give a patient personal advice. You are there to serve as part of a healthcare team assisting the patient with the management of their care, but you are not there to provide the patient with your personal insights about their condition or behavior. You may have a personal opinion about something concerning the patient, but it would not be appropriate to share that opinion with the patient the way it might be appropriate to share opinions with your friends.

Prying

Sometimes a patient may indicate that they do not want to discuss a certain topic. This is the patient's decision, and they have a right to that decision. It is inappropriate and even antagonistic for the HCP to pry into that topic once the patient has made clear that they do not want to talk about it. However, remember that prying is distinct from encouraging discussion, and an HCP with effective communication skills will understand how to strike that balance between pushing too hard on a patient and helping a patient to open up.

Becoming Defensive

Patients may at times express unhappiness or dissatisfaction with the care received, the HCP, or even the hospital or practice. The HCP should never become defensive in such cases. The HCP who becomes defensive at such times inappropriately changes the terms of the relationship from patient/provider to attacker/defender, and in such instances the therapeutic communication process, which is built on trust and understanding, completely breaks down. When a patient expresses unhappiness, the HCP should make every effort to show that they are listening carefully and empathically, and that they will attempt to address the issue making the patient unhappy.

Demanding that the Patient Explain their Behavior

The HCP should avoid demanding that the patient explain their behavior. Doing so can cause the patient to feel defensive, and when this happens the patient will no longer freely communicate with the HCP. The patient may not understand why they have acted a certain way, and to ask them for their reasons can inhibit, confuse, or even anger them. For example, the HCP should not insist that the diabetic patient who has been unable to control their eating of foods that are harmful to their blood sugar levels explain why they have been eating such foods. Rather, the HCP should focus the discussion on a plan of appropriate eating habits for a diabetic diet.

Making Commonplace, or Clichéd, Comments

In the same way that the patient deserves to feel that the HCP is giving them their undivided attention when the patient is speaking, the patient also deserves to feel that the HCP is bringing the full weight of their intelligence and thought to what they say in response to the patient. The HCP who follows up a patient history with clichés such as, *"That's the way it is sometimes,"* or *"It sounds like you're between a rock and a hard place,"* can cause the patient to feel that the HCP is just giving a mechanical, perhaps thoughtless, response. What's more, the patient could feel as if the HCP did not even listen very carefully in the first place. For example, a female patient presenting with a urinary tract infection could easily be offended by an HCP who responded to the positive urine culture results by saying, *"Well that explains the itch, doesn't it?"* A better response would be to say, *"The test results confirm our suspicion of what was causing your symptoms."*

Roadblocks to Therapeutic Communication Part II—The Patient's Behavior

Certain patient behaviors can also impede, or serve as roadblocks to, the communication process. It is important for the HCP to be on the lookout for these behaviors. Often, as in the case of certain ineffective coping behaviors, the patient is probably not even aware that they are exhibiting these. In other instances, when the patient is angry or anxious, they may or may not understand what they are communicating.

Ineffective Coping Behaviors

Patients may sometimes behave in certain ways to protect themselves from feelings of anxiety, shame, or guilt.

- Compensation—When a patient does this, they compensate, or overemphasize, a certain trait or behavior in one area because they believe they must make up for what they perceive as a deficiency, or failure, in another. For example, the middle-aged obese patient who, despite the physician's orders, does not exercise regularly or eat a healthy diet, nevertheless makes an elaborate show of telling the doctor and nurses that he has never missed a single dose of his cholesterol medicine.
- Denial—This occurs when the patient attempts, generally unconsciously, to reject or deny the existence of feelings, needs, thoughts, desires, or even facts. The cancer patient whose diagnosis has been confirmed by blood tests, x-rays, computed tomography (CT) scans, and positron emission tomography (PET) scans still thinks the doctors might have gotten it wrong. Perhaps, this patient thinks, the medical staff has mistakenly confused their tests with those of another patient.

■ Displacement—This occurs when it is impossible for the patient to accept ownership of certain thoughts, feelings, needs, or desires and attributes them, unconsciously, to a more acceptable substitute— someone or something outside of the self. The father who is deep in grief after his child receives a cancer diagnosis would naturally feel anger as part of that grief; however, he does not understand what to do with this anger and so whenever he sees his child's doctor during an appointment, he is inexplicably hostile toward the doctor.

| ROLE **PLAY** | **The Displacer** |

With a partner—with one of you playing the role of the medical assistant and the other the patient—play out the following roles:

1 **The medical assistant whose job it is to prepare the 9-year-old cancer patient for the doctor's appearance in the examination room (e.g., take vital signs, request that the patient change into a johnny).**
2 **The parent who is angry and argues with the medical assistant at every step of the preparation process.**

How does the medical assistant work with the child and their parent? What would be some appropriate and inappropriate responses that the medical assistant could give? Explain the reasons for your answers.

■ Dissociation—When this happens, the patient is attempting to disconnect the emotional significance of certain ideas or events from those ideas or events. The patient, for example, may relay an incident of childhood abuse that the HCP knows must have been painful, and yet, in the telling of the incident, the patient does not acknowledge the pain that must have been a part of the experience.
■ Identification—This occurs when the patient mimics the behavior of someone else in order to conceal their own natural behavior because they believe such behavior is inadequate. For example, a 16-year-old college tennis player has arrived at the clinic with his father, who sits impassively while the doctor explains to the young athlete that he has torn his rotator cuff, effectively ending the patient's tennis career. The boy sits stoically and with a flat affect, or facial expression, while receiving this news from the doctor. The boy's lack of an emotional reaction imitates what he believes is the correct response, taking his father's behavior as an example.
■ Projection—This happens when the patient projects onto another person or object their own feelings, as if the feelings originated in the other person or object. A patient who feels anger over some perceived inadequacy in their care may not be able to own that anger but will instead accuse the HCP of being angry.
■ Rationalization—When a patient does this, they are using false reasoning to justify inappropriate or unacceptable behavior, hoping to

make the behavior tolerable. The patient who does not comply with the physician's orders to show up for Tuesday's colonoscopy appointment may not admit that their failure to appear was because of fear but rather will change the subject and say that the HCP did not bother to ask whether the patient was free on that Tuesday.

 The Patient Who Blames the Healthcare Team for the Patient's Noncompliance

With a partner, where one of you plays the role of the HCP and the other the patient, act out the following roles:

1 **The medical assistant, who must reschedule the colonoscopy with the patient in the example above.**
2 **The patient, who blames the doctor for their failure to appear last Tuesday for the colonoscopy and is still noncommittal about showing up next Tuesday, which is the next possible opening.**

   The medical assistant wants to ensure that the patient understands when and where they should appear for the colonoscopy.

- Regression—A patient is regressing when they unconsciously return to immature, or even infantile, behaviors or thoughts. A patient may behave in this way when confronted with especially painful or difficult circumstances.
- Repression—This is when the patient simply puts out of their mind painful or difficult thoughts, feelings, ideas, or events. A patient who is confronted with a decision whether to undergo a difficult brain biopsy and then goes days without making a decision or even considering the options is repressing all thoughts of their condition.

Angry Patients

Patients can become angry for many reasons. They may believe that they have received inadequate care, been the subject of unfair treatment, or been on the receiving end of some sort of personal slight or insult. They may be angry as a result of loss of control in the face of serious illness, or they may feel frustration over the illness itself. They may be angered by the behavior of another person. Or they may just feel that they have been the victim of ineffective therapeutic communication.

As an HCP, you will need to be able to quickly identify anger in a patient. You will also need to be able to manage that anger in an appropriate manner. Some steps that can help you in dealing with an angry patient include the following:

- Learn to recognize anger. Most people can tell immediately when they are in the presence of someone who is angry. A person who speaks in a tense voice, who acts in a difficult or stubborn manner, or who rejects or ignores your attempts to communicate is likely angry.

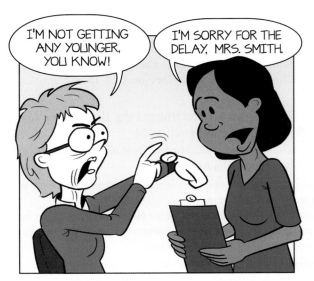

FIGURE 4-4. The Angry Patient. As an HCP, you will need to be able to quickly identify anger in a patient and then manage that anger in an appropriate manner.

- Stay calm, stay respectful, stay genuine. Your calm demeanor and respect can help to defuse anger, and your genuineness will help you to reassure the patient about addressing any concerns.
- Remember to stay focused on the patient's physical and medical needs.
- Use appropriate nonverbal communication. Maintain adequate space between yourself and the patient and keep an open posture. If possible, place yourself on the same level as the patient, standing or sitting. Maintain appropriate eye contact, but avoid staring at the patient.
- Resist the urge to defend yourself in the face of accusations from the patient. You should listen attentively to the patient and hear with an open mind what they are saying.
- Encourage the patient to be specific when describing the reasons for their anger and what they think about those reasons. Remember to demonstrate empathy to the patient by effectively paraphrasing back to them what they are telling you. Avoid simply agreeing or disagreeing with the patient. Make sure that the patient knows you understand them.
- Calmly and firmly present your point of view to the patient to help them understand what has happened. Never try to shout the patient down or do anything that would "put them in their place." This will only anger the patient more.
- Be sure to follow through completely on any promises you make in addressing the problem, and do not make any promises you cannot keep.

- Ask if the patient needs a few minutes alone to collect their thoughts and emotions.
- If you ever feel threatened by a patient's anger or you fear that a patient may do you harm, leave the room immediately and seek the help of one of the physicians or other members of the healthcare team.

Anxious Patients

Patients can be anxious for just as many reasons as they can be angry. A patient may feel anxiety just because they are present in a medical practice, the so-called "white-coat syndrome." A patient may suspect they are ill but not be sure; a patient may know they are ill; a family member or loved one may be ill.

In the same way an HCP needs to be able to recognize an angry patient, they need to be able to recognize the anxious patient. It is every bit as important to the care of the patient. Following certain steps when managing anxious patients can help.

- Quickly identify the signs of anxiety in the patient.
- Acknowledge the patient's anxiety to the patient.
- Use appropriate nonverbal communication. Maintain an appropriate distance and an open posture. Maintain appropriate eye contact. Listen attentively and empathically, making sure to effectively paraphrase what the patient tells you.
- Identify possible sources of the patient's anxiety: perhaps a procedure they are about to undergo or test results they are about to receive. A patient who recognizes that you understand the source of anxiety will more likely communicate with you.
- Make sure that the patient is as comfortable as possible physically.
- Determine what types of support the patient has, for example, family members or friends who are available and discuss those with the patient.
- Work to create a climate of warmth, acceptance, and trust. Control your own anxiety, and remain genuine and truthful.
- Never minimize or make light of the patient's anxiety, feelings, or thoughts.
- Try to help the patient cope with their anxiety by providing truthful information about the source of the anxiety.
- Notify the physician of the patient's concerns.

Communication with Other Members of the Healthcare Team—Your Colleagues

The quality of your work experience will have a lot to do with how well you communicate with the other people at work. You and your colleagues are all members of the healthcare team whose shared purpose is to provide patients with the highest level of care possible. In fulfilling that purpose, you want to use the same good communication practices with your colleagues that you would use with patients—tactfulness, courtesy, respect, empathy, genuineness, appropriate self-disclosure, and assertiveness.

Always Use an Appropriate Means of Communication with Co-Workers

There may come times when you need to resolve a dispute with a co-worker. The dispute may be purely work-related or it may have a more personal aspect. If the matter is of such a serious nature (e.g., sexual harassment, quality of patient care concerns) that a supervisor should be immediately involved, do not hesitate to involve the supervisor. If the problem is less serious, you should generally first try to reach a solution with the other party rather than involving a supervisor. There is a good chance that you and the other party will be able to resolve your differences.

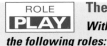 **The Dispute with Your Colleague**

With a partner, each of you playing the role of an HCP, act out the following roles:

1 **A medical assistant who consistently leaves clutter in the examination rooms so that other medical assistants in the practice must do some housekeeping each time they bring a new patient into one of the examination rooms.**
2 **The other medical assistant who gets stuck with cleaning up after your colleague.**

How do you resolve the dispute? Are you certain the other medical assistant is even aware of the inconvenience they are causing you?

For everyday matters in the medical practice, by far the most common means of communicating with others will be face-to-face. Some circumstances may call for email and others still for paper-based communication (for a full discussion of these see Chapter 9, "Electronic Communication").

The Appropriate Attitude is Assertive, not Aggressive

Maintaining an assertive yet friendly manner of communication lets others in the workplace know that you are there to do your job as effectively as possible. Understanding what you believe is right and feeling comfortable and confident in asserting that will send a signal to your co-workers that you are someone who can be counted on to work hard in the service of patient care. Most conflicts in the workplace come about through misinformation or poor communication.

Always Choose an Appropriate Time and Place for Important Communication

Remember to always be considerate of your co-workers' time. If you have an important matter to discuss with a co-worker and you believe it will take some time, show respect by asking if that co-worker has time available to make an appointment to talk.

Communication with Other Members of the Healthcare Team—Your Supervisor

How much you enjoy your job and how far you advance will have a lot to do with how effectively you communicate with your supervisor. As with patients and co-workers, you should use good communication practices.

Keep Supervisors Informed

You must recognize early on that it is very important to keep your supervisor informed when anything goes wrong. Of greatest importance is the patient, and if you ever have a concern about the quality of patient care in your practice, you must let your supervisor know—immediately. If the concern is something less serious—such as disorderly conditions in some of the examination rooms' cabinets; or even something purely office related, such as the breakdown of the copy or fax machine—you should let your supervisor know at an appropriate time. Informing your supervisor of these issues is important to the smooth running of the practice. In a larger, professional sense, though, informing your supervisor of these issues lets them know that you are someone who can be trusted to make sure that the practice is meeting patient care and workplace standards.

Ask Questions

If you are ever unsure about the right thing to do, be sure to ask. It is always better to ask a question before acting than to act without asking and make a mistake. You might fear that by asking the question you will annoy your supervisor, and it is true that repeated questions about responsibilities an employee should already have mastered can be irritating. However, the risk of annoying a supervisor by asking a question is, in most cases, smaller than the risk of annoying a supervisor by making a mistake that could have been avoided by simply asking. Finally, where patient care is concerned, you should not take any risk: If you're not sure, always ask.

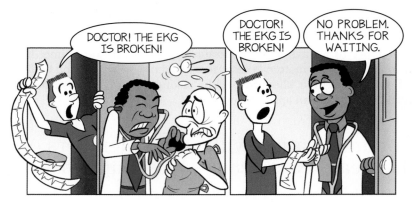

FIGURE 4-5. **Minimize Interruptions to Your Supervisor's Time.** Asking questions of your supervisor at an appropriate time can save both of you from a frustrating experience.

Minimize Interruptions of Your Supervisor's Time

You should show the same consideration to your supervisor that you show to your co-workers. If you have a matter you want to discuss with them, make the effort to make sure they have time. Ask them, "Do you have a couple of minutes to talk?" or "Is there a time I can talk to you? I have a couple of questions I want to ask." Finally, it is a good practice to save questions until you have a few you can ask at once, rather than repeatedly interrupting your supervisor during the course of a busy day. Behaving in this manner will indicate to your supervisor that you are thinking about effective professional communication practices.

Show Initiative

Keep your eyes and ears open at work. If you believe you have found a more effective or efficient way of completing some task, make it known to your supervisor in the appropriate manner. Your supervisor will appreciate your conscientiousness and will recognize in you someone who is working hard to provide the best patient care and for the good of the practice.

HIPAA—The Health Insurance Portability and Accountability Act—and Patient Privacy

HIPAA, or the Health Insurance Portability and Accountability Act, is a law that was enacted by the United States Congress in 1996. HIPAA affects every person who works in any of the health professions, so an understanding of how to comply with the law is essential.

HIPAA was initially enacted to protect workers in the United States from being denied health insurance coverage when they changed jobs. The law's authors wanted to ensure that workers' health benefits would be *portable* — that is, that workers could change jobs with the confidence that their health insurance would not have to be interrupted between jobs or at the start of the new job—as indicated by the word "portability" in the law's name. This first part of the law has come to be called Title I: Health Insurance Reform.

The second part of HIPAA, Title II: Administrative Simplification, is the portion of the law that will most directly affect you as a healthcare professional. This law contains strict requirements on the protection, maintenance, use, and electronic transfer of confidential patient data and health information.

The healthcare organization for which you work is required by part of this federal law—*The HIPAA Standards for Privacy of Individually Identifiable Health Information*, also known as the **HIPAA Privacy Rule**—to protect patients' rights by ensuring the privacy of patients' health information. Under the HIPAA Privacy Rule, your healthcare organization must:

- Have in place privacy policies and procedures that are appropriate for its healthcare services;
- Notify patients of their privacy rights and how their private health information can be used or disclosed;
- Train all employees so that they understand the privacy policies and procedures;
- Appoint a privacy official who is responsible for ensuring that the privacy policies and procedures are enforced;
- Safeguard patients' records.

Some state laws were already in place when HIPAA was enacted; these differed from the federal law in stringency, or strictness, in the protection of patients' private information. However, the federal law was written so that in any case the stricter, or more stringent, privacy protection rules—the state or federal—should apply. Your healthcare organization must have in place policies and procedures that comply with either the state or federal law, whichever is stricter.

Your healthcare organization must provide all patients with a **Notice of Privacy Practices (NPP),** stating policies and procedures by which patient health information may be disclosed. Your healthcare organization must also make a good faith effort to have the patient sign a separate document called an **Acknowledgment of Receipt of Notice of Privacy Practices,** and your organization must document in the patient's medical record whether the patient has signed this acknowledgment.

As an HCP, you will be responsible for understanding and using your organization's privacy practices. You will be responsible for protecting the confidentiality of patients' private health information.

Aside from the following small number of exceptions listed, the use and disclosure of this information are permitted only for **treatment, payment, and healthcare operations—or TPO**—and for no other reason. Specifically, TPO includes:

■ Treatment—this includes any consultation or discussion of a patient's care with other HCPs for the purposes of treating the patient;
■ Payment—this allows the healthcare organization to submit claims to health plans and insurers on behalf of patients for billing and collections;
■ Operations—this includes activities such as accreditation, employee training, and quality control.

The only exceptions to this rule include the following:

■ Court Orders—such as when a court subpoenas a patient's health information for the purposes of a criminal or civil court case;
■ Workers' Compensation Cases—such as when a workers' compensation administration board may handle insurance claims for a state;
■ Statutory Reports—such as when a state health or social services department needs this information for the purposes of protecting the general population from communicable diseases; however, state laws vary as to the reporting of individual disease cases or the patient's name;
■ Research—such as when physicians or medical researchers are conducting clinical research for the purposes of improving treatment; however, a patient's name may not be identified in any report based on this research.

Aside from the purposes of treatment, payment, and healthcare operations (TPO), you must work to ensure that the privacy of patient information is always protected. This information includes *everything* pertaining to treatment in the patient's medical record, as well as all other protected health information, such as:

■ Patient name
■ Address (including the street address, city, state, country, and ZIP code)
■ Relatives' and employers' names
■ Date of birth
■ Telephone numbers (including home, cell, and work)
■ Fax numbers
■ Email addresses (personal and work)
■ Social Security number
■ Medical record number

- Health plan beneficiary information (including names and numbers)
- Any account numbers
- Certificate or license numbers
- Serial or license plate number of any vehicle or other device
- Website address
- Fingerprints or voiceprints
- Photographic images

You can protect the privacy of patient information by understanding your healthcare organization's privacy practices and by remaining vigilant in your day-to-day interactions with colleagues, patients, family, and friends. In short, you should:

1 never discuss a patient's private information with another colleague unless your discussion pertains directly to treatment of the patient, payment for treatment services, or healthcare operations (TPO);
2 never disclose any information about one patient to another patient;
3 never tell family members about a patient's private health information;
4 never talk to your friends about any patient's private health information.

You should also be careful never to accidentally or inadvertently disclose any patient's health information. For example, suppose you need to call a patient named Mrs. Jarvis at her home phone number to discuss some information about a visit or treatment and you get Mrs. Jarvis's voicemail. In such a case, you should be careful not to inadvertently disclose any patient information to anyone else who may hear your voice message. Unless it is against the privacy policies of your healthcare organization, a good practice is to say, "This is the doctor's office for Mrs. Jarvis. Please call us back at 617-555-1212."

Other ways to remain vigilant include being aware of who may be within earshot when you need to discuss a patient's information with anyone; making sure that when you are finished accessing a patient's information on any computer that you completely log off from the program software; and keeping any papers containing patient information properly filed and put away when they are not needed by you or another member of the healthcare team.

REVIEW QUESTIONS

OBJECTIVE QUESTIONS

1 Assertiveness is an important quality to have only when dealing with patients, not co-workers. *(True or false?)*
2 Appropriate self-disclosure means to tell the patient everything about your experience that reminds you of their condition. *(True or false?)*

3 The quality you exhibit that tells others that it is the real you they perceive, and that you don't just go through the motions but show you really care about what you are doing is called _____ _____.

4 If a blood pressure monitor stops working while you are using it, you should just put it back in the drawer you took it from and not tell anyone because you will be suspected of having broken it. *(True or false?)*

5 A celebrity, such as a famous pop singer, has been admitted to one of the internal medicine wards down the hall in the hospital where you work. A good friend of yours is a big fan of this singer. You try to find out what the pop singer's medical details are on the hospital's computer system so that you can have something good to talk about when you see your friend. This is okay as long as your friend promises not to tell anyone else. *(True or false?)*

6 HIPAA stands for _____.

7 If an angry patient accuses all of the staff in your practice of giving poor patient care, it is your responsibility to stand up for your co-workers and let the patient know how wrong they are. *(True or false?)*

8 Saying "Get over it. Everyone has to do this stuff!" is not an effective way of managing a patient with anxiety. *(True or false?)*

9 If you know that a patient is receiving poor care, you should let your supervisor know immediately, regardless of the consequences to another employee. *(True or false?)*

10 Showing that you personally disapprove of a patient's relapse into smoking because you find smoking to be a dirty and dangerous habit is an effective form of therapeutic communication. *(True or false?)*

SHORT ANSWER QUESTIONS

1 Briefly explain the difference between an assertive and an aggressive style of communication.

2 List three HCP-generated roadblocks to therapeutic communication and explain why they are significant. Describe a clinical situation in which such roadblocks may occur and explain how to resolve them.

3 List three patient-generated roadblocks to therapeutic communication and explain why they are significant. Describe a clinical situation in which such roadblocks may occur and explain how to resolve them.

4 Briefly explain why providing easy reassurance to the patient may not be a good communication practice.

CLINICAL APPLICATIONS

1 A 67-year-old man with emphysema who has had to come to radiology for a chest x-ray is angry. He says he just had a chest x-ray done last week at another doctor's office and your office should have the films by now. "Clearly, all of you here are incompetent," he tells you in a nasty voice. He's angry because of the inconvenience to his life. He also says that you and the people you work with don't care how much radiation he's exposed to through the process. All of these x-rays will give him lung cancer if he doesn't get it from 30 years of smoking. Briefly explain the appropriate way to manage this angry patient.

2 A 17-year-old boy has arrived for a follow-up appointment with the urologist in your practice. The boy is here to receive the results of tests he has undergone to rule out testicular cancer. The boy is clearly ridden with anxiety and unable to interact with anyone in the practice without bursting into tears. Briefly explain the appropriate way to manage this anxious patient.

Fundamental Writing Skills

The section in the writing skills chapter you should complete at the end of Chapter 4 is Section 10-4. You can find this section on pages 214–222.

SUGGESTED FURTHER READING

1. Arford PH. Nurse-Physician Communication: An Organizational Accountability. *Nurs Econ.* 2005;23(2):72–77, 55. Retrieved April 2010 from Health Module database.
2. Batcheller J. Maximize your impact with leadership domains. *Nurs Manage.* 2007;38(8):52–53. Retrieved April 2010 from Research Library Core database.
3. Erlen JA, Jones M The patient no one liked. *Orthop Nurs.* 1999;18(4):76–79. Retrieved April 2010 from Health Module database.
4. Erlen JA. When the family asks, 'what happened?'. *Orthop Nurs.* 2000;19(6): 68–71. Retrieved November 23, 2008 from Health Module database.
5. Fallowfield L, Jenkins V. Communicating sad, bad, and difficult news in medicine. *Lancet.* 2004;363(9405):312–319. Retrieved April 2010 from Research Library Core database.
6. Faulkner A. ABC of palliative care: Communication with patients, families, and other professionals. *BMJ.* 1998;316(7125):130–132. Retrieved April 2010 from Health Module database.
7. Fix your professional image-stat! *RN.* 2007;70(12):25. Retrieved April 2010 from Research Library Core database.

8. Fuimano J. Let's target and achieve standards of excellence. *Nurs Manage.* 2004;35(3):10–11. Retrieved November 7, 2008 from Research Library Core database.

9. Garman AN, Fitz KD, Fraser MM. Communication and Relationship Management. *J Healthc Manag.* 2006;51(5):291–294. Retrieved April 2010 from Business Module database.

10. Mannahan CA. One unit's journey from hostility to respect. *Nurs Manage.* 2007;38(11):8–9. Retrieved November 7, 2008 from Research Library Core database.

11. Moss MS, Moss SZ, Rubinstein RL, Black HK. The metaphor of "family" in staff communication about dying and death. *J Gerontol B Psychol Sci SocSci.* 2003;58B(5):S290–296. Retrieved April 2010 from Research Library Core database.

12. Newby C. *HIPAA for Allied Health Careers.* New York: McGraw-Hill; 2009.

13. Roberts L, Bucksey SJ. Communicating With Patients: What Happens in Practice? *Phys Ther.* 2007;87(5):586–594. Retrieved April 2010 from Health Module database.

14. Saying what's on your mind...tactfully. *Work & Family Life.* 2008;22(4):6. Retrieved May 2010 from General Interest Module database.

15. Simms C. Stopping the word war. *Nurs Manage.* 2000;31(9):65–71. Retrieved April 2010 from Research Library Core database.

16. Truemper CM. Using scoring rubrics to facilitate assessment and evaluation of graduate-level nursing students. *J Nurs Educ.* 2004;43(12):562–564. Retrieved April 2010 from Education Module database.

17. Whitaker C. Dealing with difficult behavior. *Nursing.* 2000;30(6):82–83. Retrieved April 2010 from Health Module database.

5

INTERVIEWING TECHNIQUES

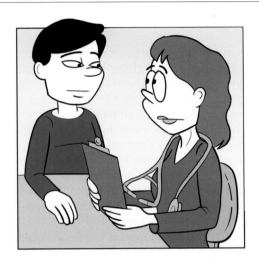

OBJECTIVES

- Understand the unequal relationship between the healthcare professional and the patient
- Describe ways in which the healthcare professional may show concern for the patient during the interview
- Determine who should be interviewed to provide medical information for a given patient
- Describe the differences between patient interviews that take place in person and those that occur over the telephone
- Distinguish between closed questions, open-ended questions, and indirect statements
- Compare and contrast the healthcare professional–centered interview and the patient-centered interview
- Understand and implement the patient interviewing guidelines
- Develop skills that lead to the "pinpointing" of the chief complaint
- Describe the legal restrictions and ethical issues associated with the patient interview

An important and fundamental step in providing medical care is the patient interview. To properly diagnose the patient's condition and to develop the appropriate treatment plan, the healthcare professional (HCP) needs to obtain a thorough and accurate medical history from the patient.

There are three primary functions of the medical interview:

■ Information gathering
■ Relationship building
■ Patient education

Each of these functions occurs to some extent during an interview. One of them may predominate in a given interview depending upon the nature of the visit; however, all three functions are essential and are dependent upon each other. Strategies for optimizing information gathering and relationship building are addressed in this chapter. Strategies for providing the patient with essential health information are discussed primarily in Chapter 7, "Patient Education."

There are two common approaches to the patient interview: the primary care provider-only approach and the team approach. In the first, primary care providers interview the patients themselves. In this way, the patient is required to relate their medical history only once. In the team approach, the patient is interviewed more than once. The first interview is conducted by a member of the healthcare team, such as a nurse or a medical assistant. This is followed by a subsequent interview conducted by the primary care provider, such as a physician, physician assistant, or nurse practitioner. Typically, a second interview is more likely to focus on the chief complaint and other critical information. Although it is more time-consuming, the team approach may result in a more thorough and complete medical record. The following discussion applies to any HCP conducting a patient interview.

A skillful HCP is adept at guiding and focusing the patient interview. As a practitioner, you must know how to encourage the best communication between yourself and your patient. This interview may be the first contact between the HCP and a patient during a particular visit. Therefore, the interview plays an important role in establishing the practitioner–patient relationship, a relationship that is based on mutual concern for the patient's well-being.

The practitioner–patient relationship is often an unequal one. Healthcare professionals are extremely knowledgeable about their area of practice and the patient is dependent upon this expertise. Therefore, it is helpful for you to equalize the relationship as much as possible. You should display an attitude of competence and professionalism and also communicate a sense of trust and confidentiality. The optimal situation is one in which the patient feels sufficiently comfortable to risk being candid about potentially sensitive topics. You can put the patient at ease even further by showing concern. A caring facial expression, an honest and genuine demeanor, and empathy will decrease the patient's feelings of anxiety and helplessness.

The Interviewee

The patient is typically the primary source of medical information; for this reason, the HCP will interview the patient directly. However, there are also instances in which the patient may be unable to provide their medical history directly to the practitioner. Patients who are critically ill or even unconscious, mentally impaired, or very young cannot effectively communicate with their caregivers. In these cases, other sources are necessary to provide the required medical information. Family members, including parents of small children and adult children of seriously ill or disoriented parents, as well as spouses and significant others, now become the primary interviewees. Finally, other healthcare team members and the medical record are excellent sources of accurate medical information regarding the patient in question.

The concept of family interviewing warrants further discussion for several reasons:

- Family members frequently accompany patients to the office visits and may serve one or more important roles
- Families are the primary context within which most health problems and illnesses occur
- The family has a powerful influence on health and illness as most health beliefs and behaviors (e.g., diet, exercise, smoking, alcohol, and drug use) are developed and maintained within the family

Family members often accompany patients to the doctor's office, the emergency room, or other clinical setting. Although some family members remain in the waiting room, many come with the patient into the examination room. This occurs most frequently when the patient is a child younger than the age of 13 years or is elderly. Sicker patients are also more likely to have family companions at their visit. Interestingly, office visits that involve other family members typically last just a few minutes longer than other visits.

The presence of family members during the visit may offer many significant benefits during the medical interview. For example, the visit may be more efficient and cost-effective because the family member can provide important information about the health problem. Furthermore, family members may:

- Help communicate the patient's concerns to the HCP
- Improve the HCP's understanding of the patient's problem
- Improve the patient's understanding of the diagnosis and treatment

- Help the patient to remember clinical information and recommendations
- Express concerns regarding the patient
- Assist the patient in making decisions

Each of these functions serves to significantly enhance the communication and understanding between the HCP and their patient.

The Setting

The interview between the HCP and the patient may take place face-to-face in the doctor's office or in a hospital or clinic. The patient interview may also take place on the telephone. These different settings have a significant influence on the way interviews are conducted.

When a patient comes to the doctor's office or to a department in the hospital, they should be escorted to an area that is both private and comfortable, usually the examination room. In this way, patient confidentiality is maintained. In a face-to-face interview, you are able to observe any nonverbal behaviors exhibited by the patient (discussed in Chapter 2). Important information such as posture, willingness to make eye contact, and physical or psychological distress may be obtained by closely observing the patient. These observations, which may be helpful in diagnosing the patient or in developing the treatment plan, should then be noted on the medical history form.

When conducting the interview on the telephone, the HCP may find it helpful to imagine that the interviewer and the interviewee are sitting back-to-back instead of face-to-face. In this case, the HCP is unable to observe the patient's facial expressions, cannot make eye contact with the patient, and is unable to receive any other visual feedback, such as body language. Instead, the practitioner conducting the interview relies on the patient's tone, pacing of speech, and word selection to interpret their condition and attitude. It is important to note that the patient will also draw conclusions regarding the interviewer based on these factors. Care must be taken to avoid misinterpretation of any kind. A cold, aloof, overly formal telephone voice will likely cause the patient to feel put-off or as if they are bothering the medical staff. A warm, welcoming telephone voice is most likely to put the patient at ease and make them feel more comfortable during the course of the interview.

Finally, the interview will proceed more smoothly if the HCP concentrates on enunciating, or carefully pronouncing, their words and on being understood by the patient. It will be very frustrating for the patient if they are repeatedly asking or saying:

"What?" or
"Can you repeat that?" or
"I can't understand you."

Types of Questions

There are two types of questions that the HCP will ask the patient during the interview: closed (direct) questions and open-ended questions.

Closed questions are designed to elicit short, focused responses such as a simple *yes* or *no*. These questions actually limit the information sought from the patient. However, the Detailed Report of Medical History Form in Figure 5-1 consists predominantly of this type of question.

		NO. OF ATTACHED SHEETS:
MEDICAL RECORD	**REPORT OF MEDICAL HISTORY**	DATE OF EXAM

NOTE: This information is for official and medically-confidential use only and will not be released to unauthorized persons

1. NAME OF PATIENT *(Last, first, middle)*   2. IDENTIFICATION NUMBER   3. GRADE

4a. HOME ADDRESS *(Street or RFD; City or Town; State; and ZIP Code)*   5. EXAMINING FACILITY

4b. CITY   4c. STATE   4d. ZIP CODE

6. PURPOSE OF EXAMINATION

7. STATEMENT OF PATIENT'S PRESENT HEALTH AND MEDICATIONS CURRENTLY USED *(Use additional pages if necessary)*

a. PRESENT HEALTH   b. CURRENT MEDICATION   REGULAR OR INTERM.

c. ALLERGIES *(Include insect bites/stings and common foods)*   d. HEIGHT   e. WEIGHT

8. PATIENT'S OCCUPATION   9. ARE YOU *(Check one)* ☐ RIGHT HANDED   ☐ LEFT HANDED

10. PAST/CURRENT MEDICAL HISTORY

CHECK EACH ITEM	YES	NO	DON'T KNOW	CHECK EACH ITEM	YES	NO	DON'T KNOW	CHECK EACH ITEM	YES	NO	DON'T KNOW
Household contact with anyone with tuberculosis				Shortness of breath				Bone, joint or other deformity			
Tuberculosis or positive TB test				Pain or pressure in chest				Loss of finger or toe			
Blood in sputum or when coughing				Chronic cough				Painful or "trick" shoulder or elbow			
				Palpitation or pounding heart				Recurrent back pain or any back injury			
Excessive bleeding after injury or dental work				Heart trouble				"Trick" or locked knee			
Suicide attempt or plans				High or low blood pressure				Foot trouble			
Sleepwalking				Cramps in your legs				Nerve injury			
Wear corrective lenses				Frequent indigestion				Paralysis *(include infantile)*			
Eye surgery to correct vision				Stomach, liver, or intestinal trouble				Epilepsy or seizure			
Lack vision in either eye				Gall bladder trouble or gallstones				Car, train, sea or air sickness			
Wear a hearing aid				Jaundice or hepatitis				Frequent trouble sleeping			
Stutter or stammer				Broken bones				Depression or excessive worry			
Wear a brace or back support				Adverse reaction to medication				Loss of memory or amnesia			
Scarlet fever				Skin diseases				Nervous trouble of any sort			
Rheumatic fever				Tumor, growth, cyst, cancer				Periods of unconsciousness			
Swollen or painful joints				Hernia				Parent/sibling with diabetes, cancer, stroke or heart disease			
Frequent or severe headaches				Hemorrhoids or rectal disease							
Dizziness or fainting spells				Frequent or painful urination				X-ray or other radiation therapy			
Eye trouble				Bed wetting since age 12				Chemotherapy			
Hearing loss				Kidney stone or blood in urine				Asbestos or toxic chemical exposure			
Recurrent ear infections				Sugar or albumin in urine							
Chronic or frequent colds				Sexually transmitted disease				Plate, pin or rod in any bone			
Severe tooth or gum trouble				Recent gain or loss of weight				Easy fatigability			
Sinusitis				Eating disorder (anorexia, bulimia, etc.)				Been told to cut down or criticized for alcohol use			
Hay Fever or allergic rhinitis				Arthritis, Rheumatism or Bursitis				Used illegal substances			
Head injury								Used tobacco			
Asthma				Thyroid trouble or goiter							

NSN 7540-00-181-8638
Previous edition not usable

STANDARD FORM 93 (REV. 6/96) (EG)
Prescribed by ICMR/GSA
FIRMR (41 CFR) 201-9.202-1
Designed using Perform Pro, WHS/DIOR, Apr 97

FIGURE 5-1. Detailed Report of Medical History Form. (*continued*)

11. FEMALES ONLY						
CHECK EACH ITEM	YES	NO	DON'T KNOW	DATE OF LAST MENSTRUAL PERIOD	DATE OF LAST PAP SMEAR	DATE OF LAST MAMMO-GRAM
Treated for a female disorder						
Change in menstrual pattern						

CHECK EACH ITEM. IF "YES" EXPLAIN IN BLANK SPACE TO RIGHT. LIST EXPLANATION BY ITEM NUMBER.		
ITEM	YES	NO
12. Have you been refused employment or been unable to hold a job or stay in school because of:		
a. Sensitivity to chemicals, dust, sunlight, etc.		
b. Inability to perform certain motions.		
c. Inability to assume certain positions.		
d. Other medical reasons (If yes, give reasons.)		
13. Have you ever been treated for a mental condition? (If yes, specify when, where, and give details.)		
14. Have you ever been denied life insurance? (If yes, state reason and give details.)		
15. Have you had, or have you been advised to have, any operation? (If yes, describe and give age at which occurred.)		
16. Have you ever been a patient in any type of hospital? (If yes, specify when, where, why, and name of doctor and complete address of hospital.)		
17. Have you consulted or been treated by clinics, physicians, healers, or other practitioners within the past 5 years for other than minor illnesses? (If yes, give complete address of doctor, hospital, clinic, and details.)		
18. Have you ever been rejected for military service because of physical, mental, or other reasons? (If yes, give date and reason for rejection.)		
19. Have you ever been discharged from military service because of physical, mental, or other reasons? (If yes, give date, reason, and type of discharge; whether honorable, other than honorable, for unfitness or unsuitability.)		
20. Have you ever received, is there pending, or have you ever applied for pension or compensation for existing disability? (If yes, specify what kind, granted by whom, and what amount, when, why.)		
21. Have you ever been arrested or convicted of a crime, other than minor traffic violations? (If yes, provide details.)		
22. Have you ever been diagnosed with a learning disability? (If yes, give type, where, and how diagnosed.)		
23. LIST ALL IMMUNIZATIONS RECEIVED		

I certify that I have reviewed the foregoing information supplied by me and that it is true and complete to the best of my knowledge. I authorize any of the doctors, hospitals, or clinics mentioned above to furnish the Government a complete transcript of my medical record for purposes of processing my application for this employment or service. I understand that falsification of information on Government forms is punishable by fine and/or imprisonment.

24a. TYPED OR PRINTED NAME OF EXAMINEE	24b. SIGNATURE	24c. DATE

NOTE: HAND TO THE DOCTOR OR NURSE, OR IF MAILED MARK ENVELOPE "TO BE OPENED BY MEDICAL OFFICER ONLY."

25. PHYSICIAN'S SUMMARY AND ELABORATION OF ALL PERTINENT DATA (Physician shall comment on all positive answers in items 7 through 11. Physician may develop by interview any additional medical history deemed important, and record any significant findings here.)

26a. TYPED OR PRINTED NAME OF PHYSICIAN OR EXAMINER	26b. SIGNATURE	26c. DATE

STANDARD FORM 93 (REV. 6-96) **BACK**

FIGURE 5-1. (*Continued*)

"Have you ever had rheumatic fever?"
"Have you ever had jaundice or hepatitis?"
"Do you use tobacco?"

Other examples of closed questions that the HCP may ask the patient during an interview include the following:

"Are you taking your medication as directed?"
"Do you feel nauseous now?"

"Where does it hurt?"
"Did you have a fever this morning?"
"You said that you have had high blood pressure for the past 3 years, correct?"
"Are you available for an ultrasound on Thursday?"

Closed questions quickly provide a great deal of objective information about the patient. The HCP will often have only 15 minutes with the patient, and these questions will allow for the most efficient communication.

Conversely, much important information, both objective and subjective, regarding the current physical and emotional conditions of the patient can be obtained only by way of open-ended questions. These questions often begin with *who, what, where, when, how,* and *why.* As such, open-ended questions cannot be answered simply and require more discussion regarding a given health issue. These are the questions that help to establish therapeutic communication and a relationship between the patient and the HCP. The patient is required to provide more explanation when responding to these questions. Furthermore, the HCP has the opportunity to paraphrase the patient's response and empathize with the patient.

Open-ended questions often begin with *how* or *what.* Examples of these questions include the following:

"How are your stress levels at work?"
"How has the new medication affected your sleep?"
"What does this pain feel like?"
"What conditions bring on an attack of angina?"
"What did the doctor tell you about taking these medications?"

Open-ended statements may also be useful.

"Describe when this occurs."
"Give me an example."

The use of questions beginning with *why* should be used with caution. Consider the following questions:

"Why don't you take your medication?"
"Why did you do that?"

There may be no one true answer to a *why* question, as a patient's motivation is often complex. In addition, these questions may be perceived as confrontational. The patient may feel as though they have to defend themselves, and this is likely to inhibit further communication and damage the therapeutic relationship between the practitioner and the patient.

On the other hand, there are times when "why" questions are useful. For example, to engage in true collaborative decision making, it is necessary for the HCP to know what motivates the patient. The HCP will often need to ask the patient about the factors that might influence their ability to follow a certain treatment regimen. Consider the following questions:

"Why are you concerned about taking this medication?'
"Why are you worried about beginning this diet?"
"Why do you think that is?"

In these situations, the questions are meant to improve the HCP's understanding of how the patient feels about the given issue. Better understanding between the HCP and the patient often leads to enhanced patient compliance and improved health outcomes.

The use of *leading* questions and statements should be avoided. Such questions could include:

"You haven't had heart palpitations, have you?"
"I assume you have shortness of breath."

These types of questions or statements are likely to prompt or encourage the patient to provide what they perceive is the desired answer. If the patient does not fully understand the content of the question, they may be compelled to simply go along with the HCP to avoid appearing disagreeable. These responses may, in fact, be inaccurate and have a negative impact on the medical interview.

Another technique that may be employed during the patient interview involves the use of indirect statements. As with open-ended questions, these types of statements help to establish therapeutic communication and a relationship between the practitioner and the patient. An additional advantage to such statements involves obtaining information from the patient without the patient feeling questioned. Examples of indirect statements include the following:

"Tell me about the diet you are on."
"That must be very difficult for you."
"Tell me how the new job is going."
"I would like to know more about these headaches you have been getting."

In addition to the section including "yes or no" questions, the Detailed Report of Medical History also has a section where explanations to various questions may be noted. Examples of these questions include the following:

"Have you ever been a patient in any type of hospital? (If yes, specify when, where, why, and name of doctor and complete address of the hospital.)"
"Have you ever been denied life insurance? (If yes, state the reason and give details.)"

Finally, there is a section in the Detailed Report of Medical History for summary and elaboration of all pertinent data. As indicated in section #25 of Figure 5-1, the HCP "may develop by interview any additional medical history deemed important, and record any significant findings here."

The HCP-centered Interview versus the Patient-centered Interview

Consider the following interview between a healthcare professional and their patient:

HCP: "What brings you here today?"
Patient: "I have chest pain."
HCP: "How severe is it?" "When does it occur?" "What do you do to relieve it?"

This is an example of the HCP-centered interview where the healthcare provider controls the dialog. The stream of questions in response to the patient's first complaint may, in fact, interrupt the patient. Interrupting the patient about the first complaint, which may not necessarily be the chief complaint, may prevent the patient from continuing to express all of their concerns.

Contrast the previous interview with the following interview:

HCP: "What brings you here today?"
Patient: "I have chest pain."

HCP: "What else?"
Patient: "I have been having a lot of trouble sleeping."

HCP: "Anything else?"
Patient: "Well, I have been very worried about my job. I am afraid that I may be laid off."

This is an example of the patient-centered interview where the HCP uses "continuers," expressions that encourage the patient to reveal all of their concerns at the beginning of the interview. The HCP allows the patient to tell their story and guides the patient to provide the important details by using both open-ended questions and indirect statements as well as specific closed questions. This approach provides the best information.

The use of continuers also contributes to the development of a relationship between the HCP and their patient at the outset of their interaction. For example, the HCP may offer an expression of empathy and concern such as "You seem very worried" or "You appear quite upset." This acknowledges the patient's feelings and encourages the patient to reveal more information.

Finally, the patient-centered approach allows the HCP to be more attentive to the nonverbal messages expressed by the patient. As discussed in Chapter 2, the patient's nonverbal behaviors, including eye contact, posture, and facial expressions, may provide important information regarding their physical and emotional state.

REPORT OF MEDICAL HISTORY
Name: _____ Date: _____
Address: _____ Phone: _____
Age: _____ Sex: _____ Marital Status: _____ Occupation: _____
Primary Care Physician: _____ Phone: _____
Complaints: _____
History: _____
Vital Signs Pulse: _____ Temp: _____ Resp: _____ BP: _____
Physical Findings: _____
Lab Tests: _____
Diagnosis: _____
Treatment: _____
Remarks: _____

FIGURE 5-2. Basic Report of Medical History Form.

Furthermore, the American Academy on Physician and Patient suggests the use of "PEARLS" during the patient-centered interview, as it contributes to the relationship-building aspect of the medical interview.

Partnership: conveys that the HCP and the patient are in this together

Empathy: expresses understanding and concern for the patient

Apology: acknowledges that the HCP is sorry that the patient had to wait, that the procedure was painful, that the lab tests will take several days to process, and so on

Respect: acknowledges the patient's suffering, anxiety, fear, and so on

Legitimization: acknowledges that the patient may be angry, frustrated, depressed, and so on

Support: conveys that the HCP will be there for the patient and not abandon them

Interviewing Guidelines

Some important guidelines, strategies, and techniques that the HCP may employ to conduct a comfortable and effective interview are outlined in this section. Where appropriate, the rationale behind a given strategy and examples for implementation of the strategy are provided. Examples of Report of Medical History Forms are found in Figures 5-1 and 5-2.

  1 *Call the patient by name.* This will not only verify that you are interviewing the intended patient, but it will also begin to establish a connection between you and the patient. Refer to the patient formally. In

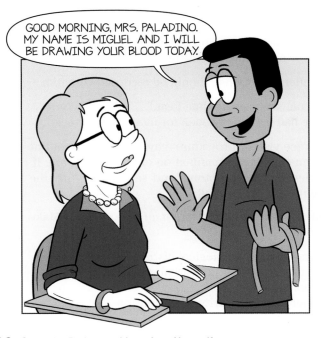

FIGURE 5-3. Greet the Patient and Introduce Yourself.

other words, use "Mr.," "Mrs.," or "Ms." First names should be used only with the patient's permission.

2 *Introduce yourself.* Tell the patient about your role in this setting and clarify the reason for the interview. Explain the procedure (e.g., routine check-up, ultrasound, electrocardiogram, pulmonary function test, cardiac stress test) and its purpose to the patient.

3 *Show concern for the patient.* A warm, caring facial expression; honest, genuine responses; and empathy will help the patient to feel comfortable during the interview. The more comfortable the patient feels, the more forthcoming they will be when responding to your questions.

4 *Convey an attitude of competence and professionalism.* The proper attitude, as well as the proper attire, will help to put the patient at ease and help to establish the patient's trust in you as a healthcare professional.

5 *Sit opposite the patient.* The interviewer should sit approximately an arm's length from the patient and maintain a relaxed but attentive posture. This arrangement will allow you to establish eye contact with the patient and to make visual observations for notation in the medical record. Eye contact is an important aspect in establishing a connection between the interviewer and the interviewee.

6 *Ask about the chief complaint first.* This will provide an indication as to why the patient has come to seek medical attention.

"How have you been feeling since your last office visit?"
"What seems to be the problem?"
"What brings you to see the doctor today?"

The patient's response should be recorded verbatim.

"I feel nauseous every time I eat."
"I have had pain in my back for more than a week."

The office visit or procedure may, in fact, be a routine one, such as an annual physical examination or a mammogram. If the patient is experiencing no symptoms and says *I feel fine*, the HCP should make note of this as well.

7 *Perform a visual assessment of the patient.* Make note of any observations, including:

■ Physical or psychological distress of the patient
■ Posture and other nonverbal signals
■ Grooming
■ Coherence and clarity of expression

Body language often conveys a message of its own. For example, a patient who is upset physically or emotionally may not make eye

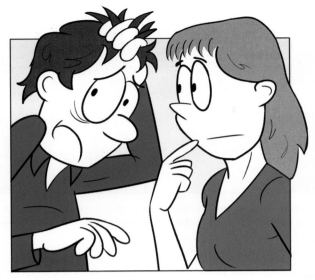

FIGURE 5-4. Visual Assessment. Visual assessment of the patient allows the HCP to make note of physical or psychological distress as well as any forms of nonverbal communication.

contact with you or they may sit with their arms crossed tightly. There may be times when the patient's nonverbal communication conflicts with their verbal communication. In this instance, you may find it helpful to make this observation to the patient in an effort to draw them out and to encourage them to be more forthcoming.

8 *Be nonjudgmental.* Never pass judgment or condemn a patient for their healthcare practices or beliefs. Negative feedback to a patient's statement may inhibit further openness. The patient may now be less likely to reveal other important or relevant information. Positive feedback may cause the patient to lose focus and discuss topics that are not relevant to the chief complaint or the question at hand.

9 *Use short probing questions.* Speak slowly, clearly, and distinctly. Direct questions will help to eliminate ambiguous responses or confusion on the part of the patient. A direct question is more likely to result in a direct answer.

"How often does this occur?"
"Can you point to where it hurts?"
"When did you notice that you were losing weight?"

10 *Use simple questions and statements that the patient will understand.* Healthcare professionals must communicate effectively and

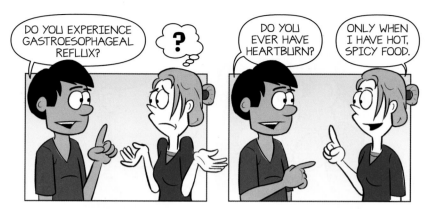

FIGURE 5-5. Simple Questions. The use of simple questions and statements, as well as common terms instead of medical terms, will facilitate the communication between the HCP and their patient.

professionally with their colleagues as well as their patients. When communicating with colleagues, it is appropriate to use clinical terms as they are more accurate and informative. However, you should remember that most patients are unfamiliar with medical terminology and the language associated with a given medical specialty. During the interview, you should use terminology that the patient will understand. A patient cannot provide accurate responses to questions they cannot comprehend.

Example: "Describe the nature of your gastrointestinal distress."
Better: "Do you have nausea, vomiting, or diarrhea?"

Example: "How long have you been experiencing amenorrhea?"
Better: "When was your last period?"

 ROLE   **Using Simple Questions and Statements**
PLAY   *With a partner, identify better ways of expressing the following messages to a patient:*

a. The insulin will help you to avoid hyperglycemia.
b. Do you experience vertigo when you stand up too fast after lying down?
c. This diuretic is for your hypertension.
d. Osteoporosis is more prevalent in older women.
e. The cause of your dyspnea is the pulmonary embolism.
f. Your father has had a cerebrovascular accident.
g. Your baby has bilateral otitis again.
h. How long have you been experiencing this pharyngitis?
i. The burning you feel when you urinate may be due to nephritis.
j. This cancer treatment is likely to cause alopecia.

11 *Give the patient time to answer fully before going on to the next question.* Many individuals think out loud. The patient needs to fully process the question and then determine how they really want to answer it. As such, the true answer to the question may change over the course of the response. The practitioner should always be efficient; however, the patient should never feel rushed.

12 *Listen attentively and respond with interest.* This is perhaps one of the most important aspects of effective communication. Listening is not simply hearing words. It also involves being attentive to the way the words are actually said by the patient. In other words, the HCP must strive to understand the feelings underlying the spoken word.

Another important aspect of listening is being aware of what the patient has left out of their verbal response. This may also provide important information regarding the patient's feelings. The HCP should be entirely focused on the patient and listen closely to all responses. In this way, the interviewer will be able to record the most accurate facts and information. The occasional brief silence can slow the pace of the interview, allow you to make notations in the health record, and may also allow the patient to elaborate on their response.

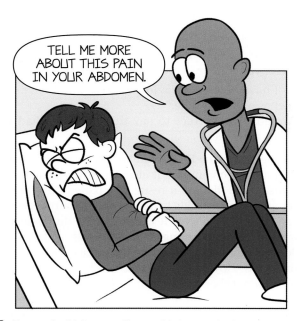

FIGURE 5-6. Respond with Interest. Expressing interest in the patient's message helps to maximize the patient's verbal responses and to achieve a full understanding of the patient's feelings.

Interest may be established by making encouraging or prompting statements.

"That's quite interesting."
"Could you explain that more fully?"
"And then what happens?"

In this way, you will help to maximize the patient's verbal responses.

13 *Use continuers.* The physical set-up of the interview area is often highly organized and efficient. In such an environment, patients may feel compelled to answer questions as briefly and concisely as possible. However, these responses may not provide all of the necessary information regarding their condition. As discussed previously, the use of "continuers" may also help to draw out the patient and encourage them to elaborate. Examples of continuers include:

"What else?"
"Anything else?"

These expressions may allow the patient to reveal all of their thoughts and concerns. They may also allow the patient to verbalize their true chief complaint earlier in the interview.

14 *Paraphrase important statements.* Information recorded during the patient interview must be as accurate as possible. A helpful technique in achieving accuracy is repeating the information.

Patient: "I get chest pains whenever I go up the stairs in my house."
HCP: "Tell me if I have it right that you get chest pains whenever you exert yourself or exercise?"

Patient: "I have been under a lot of stress and I have been getting headaches all of the time."
HCP: "Would it be correct to say that you have had a headache every day this week?"

Paraphrasing allows the HCP to immediately verify their understanding of the patient's comments. It also allows the patient to hear what their words sound like. As a result, the patient may want to clarify what they said. Paraphrasing helps to build rapport between the interviewer and the interviewee. It confirms that the patient is actually being listened to. Paraphrasing maintains focus on the patient. Finally, it may keep the patient talking and encourage them to elaborate on their comments. However, you must be careful not to overuse this technique as it may become irritating to the patient.

15 *Seek clarification.* It is often helpful for the HCP to gently probe the patient and encourage them to offer further information.

"I'm not sure what you mean."
"I don't think I fully understand what you are saying."

In fact, at times it may be necessary to interrupt the patient. This will allow you to clarify important points and to slow down the interview process so that all relevant information can be accurately assessed and recorded.

"How often does that occur?"
"Could you describe that feeling more specifically?"
"Where is the pain?"

As with paraphrasing, this verbal feedback reassures the patient that you are listening closely.

 Paraphrasing and Seeking Clarification
With a partner—one of you as patient and one as HCP—act out each of the following scenarios in which the patient presents a complaint and the HCP paraphrases it back. If the patient is ambiguous, the HCP should seek clarification.

a. **Henry is an 83-year-old man who complains to his wife Margaret about severe chest pain. Very concerned, his wife calls for an ambulance. Upon arrival at Henry's home, the paramedic has a brief discussion with Henry about his symptoms.**
b. **Annie is a nutritionist at a nearby healthcare center. Her first patient of the day is an obese male high school sophomore. The goal of this visit is to assess his dietary patterns.**

Discuss how these techniques enhanced the communication between the patient and the HCP. What clarification and further information was obtained as a result?

---

16 *Verbalize the implied.* Patients may not always express themselves directly. In this case, the HCP will have to infer, or derive a conclusion about, what the patient really means. To avoid potentially inaccurate interpretation of the patient's statement, you may encourage the patient to be specific by offering a follow-up statement or question.

Patient: "My high blood pressure is probably due to my new boss."
HCP: "Why is it due to your new boss?"

Patient: "I have not been exercising."
HCP: "Can you explain why not? How does exercising affect your asthma?"

17 *Avoid getting off the subject.* The interview should remain focused on the patient and their medical information. Wandering off onto other topics is inappropriate, unprofessional, and wastes valuable time. However, there may be instances where patients need to vent and express their feelings.

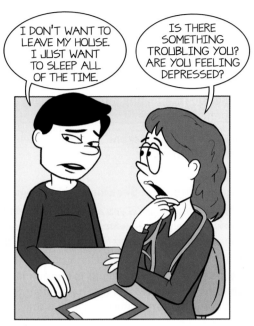

FIGURE 5-7. Verbalize the Implied. The patient may not express himself directly. In this case, the HCP will have to infer, or derive a conclusion about, what the patient really means.

18 *Introduce additional questions.* The presence of some diseases such as HIV and hepatitis B may require the HCP to ask further questions of the patient regarding any history of illicit intravenous drug use and their sexual activity. All delicate subjects should be handled with the highest level of tact and delicacy. Once again, you should avoid being judgmental and should remain professional at all times.

19 *Utilize the section for comments in the Medical History Forms.* These forms often have a section for additional comments (Figures 5-1 and 5-2). This space may be used by the HCP to document any other important information (e.g., race, age, loss of a loved one, or other stress-inducing life events). Certain races, ages, and genders have a higher disposition for certain diseases or disorders. For example, hypertension, or high blood pressure, is more prevalent in blacks than in whites. Ear infections are more prevalent in children between 6 and 20 months of age than in children older than 6 years of age. Anemia, osteoporosis, and urinary tract infections are more prevalent in women than in men. Finally, the patient may not realize that personal information may be relevant and further explanation may be recorded here.

TABLE 5-1

Summary of Interviewing Guidelines

- Call the patient by name.
- Introduce yourself.
- Show concern for the patient.
- Convey an attitude of competence and professionalism.
- Sit opposite the patient.
- Ask about the chief complaint first.
- Perform a visual assessment of the patient.
- Be nonjudgmental.
- Use short probing questions.
- Use simple questions and statements that the patient will understand.
- Give the patient time to answer fully before going on to the next question.
- Listen attentively and respond with interest.
- Use continuers.
- Paraphrase important statements.
- Seek clarification.
- Verbalize the implied.
- Avoid getting off subject.
- Introduce additional questions.
- Utilize the section for comments in the medical history forms.
- Immediately record the information.
- Summarize.
- Thank the patient.

20 *Immediately record the information.* The HCP should immediately record patient information obtained during the interview. This will ensure an accurate and complete medical history and eliminate the need for you to rely on memory.

21 *Summarize.* A summary at the end of the interview allows the HCP to verify the accuracy and the completeness of the medical history.

22 *Thank the patient.* When the interview has come to a close, the HCP should provide the patient with an opportunity to ask any questions. This is followed with an explanation of the next step in the examination or procedure. Finally, thank the patient. (See "Summary of Interviewing Guidelines" in Table 5-1)

Pinpointing the Chief Complaint or Present Illness

A primary goal of the interview is to identify the patient's chief complaint. Questioning the patient during the interview should focus on, or pinpoint, specific symptoms or important medical information that will facilitate reaching an accurate diagnosis. This is accomplished by converting vague, general statements into clear, precise statements. The HCP needs to encourage the patient to be specific and accurate. Quantified descriptions and statements are far more useful than those that are qualified.

Example: "My knee has been hurting forever."
Pinpointed: "I have had mild pain in my knee for the past 2 months."

Example: "I always have headaches."
Pinpointed: "I have had three severe headaches this week."

Example: "My stomach never feels right."
Pinpointed: "I feel nauseous after I drink milk."

Encouraging the patient to pinpoint their symptoms promotes your understanding of the nature and the severity of the problem.

> **ROLE PLAY** **Pinpointing**
> *With a partner, identify questions or statements that will lead the patient to pinpoint their complaint for each of the preceding examples. Continue this exercise with your partner taking turns playing the patient and the HCP. The patient makes a vague statement regarding their health issue and the HCP pinpoints the problem.*

Interviewing Children and Adolescents

There are many similarities between adult patient interviews and those of children and adolescents. For example, the basic organization of the medical history and the professional guidelines for the interview are the same. Clearly, the demonstration of empathy and respect is equally important with all patients. However, there are also many differences between adult patient interviews and those of children and adolescents. These differences are based upon the stage of physical, psychological, and emotional development of the patients as they progress from infants and toddlers to school-age children and, finally, to adolescents. Throughout these stages, the patient has increasing ability to contribute to their own story.

- Infants and toddlers: Although the patient is the focus of the interview, they are usually not a participant. The patient's parent or guardian typically provides most of the information during the interview. However, it is helpful to have the child present to prompt the parent's recall of relevant details.
- School-age children: Many children are able to contribute substantially to the patient interview by the age of 5 or 6 years. However, it is important to verify the accuracy of the information with the child's parent or guardian.

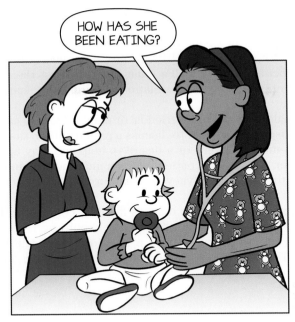

FIGURE 5-8. Infants and Toddlers. Although the very young patient is the focus of the interview, they are usually not a participant. The patient's parent or guardian typically provides most of the information during the interview.

■ Adolescents: As patients advance through their teenage years, they often begin taking increasing responsibility for their own health and health care while their parent's roles begin to diminish. These changing roles may be awkward for both the patients and their parents. Assure the adolescent that your conversation is confidential. Information regarding drug and alcohol use, sexuality, and behavioral and emotional issues should be obtained directly from the adolescent. Finally, it is helpful to avoid closed questions that would tend to elicit brief responses and perhaps, as a result, even silence.

Legal Restrictions and Ethical Issues

The most important issue involved with obtaining and recording medical information is confidentiality, or the patient's right to privacy. Face-to-face interviews are always conducted in private areas. Telephone interviews are also conducted with the utmost discretion. Medical information obtained in these interviews should not be discussed in the open office or elsewhere with family or friends or with other patients. Violations of confidentiality damage the trust between the patient and the HCP. Furthermore, these violations open practitioners to lawsuits. The Health Insurance Portability and Accountability Act of 1996 (HIPAA, discussed in Chapter 4) addresses the security and privacy issues of health data. Under HIPAA rules, covered entities, including hospitals, doctors, and all HCPs must guard against the misuse of a patient's identifiable health information and limit the sharing of such information.

Individuals such as family, friends, or employers may call the office or engage hospital personnel to discuss a patient. Often their questions are out of genuine concern or a desire to help and may appear harmless. However, discussing a patient with an unauthorized individual is a violation of the patient's privacy and can turn into an ethical and legal issue.

When calling a patient to discuss medical conditions, treatment, or finances, the patient's right to privacy should be respected at all times. Calls should be made from a location where the HCP is not overheard. The HCP should speak only with the patient, not a family member.

 ROLE PLAY   **Patient Confidentiality**

It was an October afternoon in New England. In the emergency room (ER) at a major teaching hospital in Boston, the staff members were listening to the Patriot's football game against the New York Jets. In the third quarter, one of the Jets' Pro-Bowl linemen was badly injured while making a crushing tackle. He fell to the ground and was unable to move. Fearing a spinal cord injury, emergency medical personnel immobilized him with a collar and a backboard. He was removed from the field on a cart and rushed to the hospital. Even before his ambulance pulled into the emergency entrance, television crews and newspaper reporters crowded into the ER and began asking questions.

In a small group, act out each of the following scenarios that may arise with regard to patient confidentiality. Jessica is the Director of the Emergency Department. Rob is the radiology technologist who performed the magnetic resonance imaging (MRI) on the player.

1 Mike is a reporter from a Boston newspaper who wants the details of the MRI. How should Jessica and Rob respond to Mike?

2 After the game, the head coach for the Jets arrives at the hospital and wants the details of the MRI. How should Rob respond to the coach?

3 That evening, the player's wife arrives from New York and speaks to Jessica. What should Jessica tell her?

For each of the above, refer to the previous discussion as well as the discussion on HIPAA in Chapter 4, for more details.

REVIEW QUESTIONS

OBJECTIVE QUESTIONS

1 The interviewer should sit approximately an arm's length from the patient. *(True or false?)*

2 The interviewer should avoid making eye contact with the patient and focus entirely on the medical history form in order to eliminate any mistakes in the record. *(True or false?)*

3 The patient's response should be recorded verbatim. *(True or false?)*

4 The interviewer should ask about the chief complaint first. *(True or false?)*

5 The use of complex medical terminology is recommended during the interview as it is more professional. *(True or false?)*

6 If a patient is not at home, the HCP may leave a detailed telephone message only with a family member. *(True or false?)*

7 The best open-ended questions begin with *why. (True or false?)*

SHORT ANSWER QUESTIONS

1 What are the three primary functions of the medical interview?

2 Distinguish between the primary care provider–only approach and the team approach to patient interviews.

3 What factors help to optimize the practitioner–patient relationship?

4 List potential sources of medical information other than the patient.

5 Explain how family members may enhance the communication between the HCP and their patient.

6 Explain how a telephone interview differs from a face-to-face interview. What communication issues affect the outcome of this type of interview?

7 A 55-year-old man comes to the emergency room complaining of recurring chest pain. Provide examples of closed questions, open-ended questions, and indirect statements that may be employed during the patient interview to facilitate the determination of a diagnosis.

8 Referring to the previous question regarding the patient with chest pain, what types of observations may be noted on the medical history form?

9 Discuss the benefits of paraphrasing important statements made by a patient. Provide an example of a paraphrased statement for the patient in question 7.

10 What is pinpointing? How is it accomplished? What types of questions or statements could be made to pinpoint the chief complaint for the patient in question 7?

11 Using a copy of the Report of Medical History Form in Figure 5-1, obtain a medical history from a "patient" (classmate, friend, family member).

Clinical Applications

1 An 87-year-old man has arrived for his annual check-up. As you conduct the patient interview, he begins telling you stories about his late wife and his four grandchildren. Each question you ask elicits another story. Describe the techniques you should employ for guiding the interview and to gently help the patient to focus and stay on track.

2 A 5-year-old boy has come to the emergency room with a complaint of abdominal pain. However, he is not communicative and he either does not talk or he answers your questions with only a word or two. Describe the techniques you should employ to open him up and obtain the information you need. If these techniques are unsuccessful, what other methods may help you to obtain relevant information regarding this patient?

Fundamental Writing Skills

The section in the writing skills chapter you should complete at the end of Chapter 5 is Section 10-5. You can find this section on pages 222–226.

SUGGESTED FURTHER READING

1. Abou-Auda HS. Communication Skills. Retrieved April 2010 from http://faculty.ksu.edu.sa/hisham/Documents/PHCL455/Communication_Skills_Hisham.pdf.
2. Adams CH, Jones PD. *Interpersonal Communication Skills for Health Professionals.* 2nd ed. Glencoe McGraw-Hill: New York; 2000.
3. Barrier PA, Li JTC, Jensen NM. Two words to improve physician-patient communication: what else? *Mayo Clin Proc.* 2003;78:211–214.
4. Beck RS, Daughtridge R, Sloane PD. Physician-patient communication in the primary care office: a systematic review. *J Am Board Fam Pract.* 2002;15: 25–38.
5. Beckman HB, Frankel RM. The effect of physician behavior on the collection of data. *Ann Intern Med.* 1984;101:692–696.
6. Campbell TL. The family's impact on health: a critical review and annotated bibliography. *Fam Syst Med.* 1986;4(2 & 3):135–328.
7. Campbell TL, Patterson JM. The effectiveness of family interventions in the treatment of physical illness. *J Marital Fam Ther.* 1995;21(4):545–583.

8. Campbell TL, McDaniel SH, Cole-Kelly K, et al. Family interviewing: a review of the literature in primary care. *Fam Med.* 2002;34(5):312–318.

9. Cole-Kelly K, Yanoshik MK, Campbell J, et al. Integrating the family into routine patient care: a qualitative study. *J Fam Pract.* 1998;47(6):440–445.

10. Coulehan JL, Block ML. *The Medical Interview, Mastering Skills for Clinical Practice.* 5th ed. Philadelphia: FA Davis Co; 2006.

11. Doherty WA, Campbell TL. *Families and Health.* Beverly Hills, CA: Sage Press; 1988.

12. Everitt K. Good Patient Communication May Prevent Medical Errors. 2007. Retrieved April 2010 from www.sfc-acs.org/information/GoodPatientCommunicationMayPreventMedicalErrors.doc.

13. Freeman R. Communicating effectively: some practical suggestions. *Br Dent J.* 1999;187(5).

14. Frew MA. *Comprehensive Medical Assisting: Competencies for Administrative and Clinical Practice,* 3rd ed. Philadelphia: FA Davis Co; 1995.

15. House JS, Landis KR, Umberson D. Social relationships and health. *Sci.* 1988;241(4865):540–545.

16. http://www.brooksidepress.org/Products/OperationalMedicine/DATA/operationalmed/Forms/sf0093.pdf. Retrieved April 2010.

17. Keir L, Wise BA, Krebs C. *Medical Assisting, Administrative and Clinical Competencies,* 5th ed. Clifton Park, NY: Thomson Delmar Learning; 2003.

18. Lazare A, Putnam SM, Lipkin M. Three Functions of the Medical Interview. In: Lipkin M, Putnam SM, Lazare A, eds. *The Medical Interview: Clinical Care Education and Research.* New York: Springer-Verlag; 1995.

19. Lindh WQ, Pooler MS, Tamparo CD, et al. *Comprehensive Medical Assisting, Administrative and Clinical Competencies.* 4th ed. Clifton Park, NY: Thomson Delmar Learning; 2009.

20. Lussier MT, Richard C. Doctor-patient communication, the medical interview. *Can Fam Physician.* 2004. Retrieved April 2010 from http://www.cfpc.ca/cfp/2004/Jan/vol50-jan-clinical-4.asp.

21. Marvel MK, Morphew PK. Levels of family involvement by resident and attending physicians. *Fam Med.* 1993;25(1):26–30.

22. Medalie JH, Zyzanski SJ, Langa D, et al. The family in family practice: is it a reality? *J Fam Pract.* 1998;46(5):390–396.

23. Scatena L, Schilling L, Lin C, et al. Companions Accompanying Patients to Internal Medicine Ambulatory Visits: Characteristics and Rationales. Presented at the 1999 Society of General Internal Medicine Annual Conference in Washington, D.C.

6

ADAPTING COMMUNICATION TO A PATIENT'S ABILITY TO UNDERSTAND

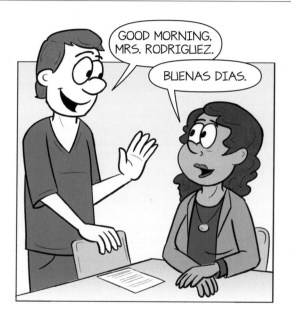

OBJECTIVES

- Explain how low health literacy may impact a patient's health
- Describe several strategies that will facilitate communication between a healthcare professional and a patient with low health literacy
- Explain how language barriers may impact communication between a healthcare professional and their patient
- Describe several strategies that will facilitate communication between a healthcare professional and a patient who speaks a different language
- Describe several strategies that will facilitate communication between a healthcare professional and a patient who is visually impaired
- Describe several strategies that will facilitate communication between a healthcare professional and a patient who is deaf or hard of hearing

■ Explain how advanced age may impact communication between a healthcare professional and their patient
■ Describe several strategies that will facilitate communication between a healthcare professional and an elderly patient
■ Distinguish between delirium and dementia
■ Describe several strategies that will facilitate communication between a healthcare professional and a patient with impaired cognitive abilities

As discussed in previous chapters, pain, fear, and anxiety may negatively impact communication with any patient. Moreover, low health literacy, language differences, visual impairment, loss of hearing, advanced age, or confusion may also impair communication in some patients. Therefore, healthcare professionals (HCPs) must learn to adapt their communication for these patients in order to remain effective when delivering their message. This chapter discusses strategies that will enable the HCP to enhance communication with their patients under these specialized circumstances. It is important to note that these additional insights and skills may be applicable to all patients.

Health Literacy

In its *Healthy People 2010* report, the U.S. Department of Health and Human Services defines health literacy as "the degree to which individuals have the capacity to obtain, process, and understand basic health information and services needed to make appropriate health decisions." Health literacy includes the ability to understand instructions on over-the-counter and prescription drug labels, appointment slips, medical education brochures, doctor's instructions, and consent forms, as well as the ability to navigate complex healthcare systems. Most consent forms, insurance forms, and medication package inserts are written at a high school reading level or higher. However, over time most individuals' reading abilities fall three to five grade levels below the last year of school completed. Therefore, people with a high school diploma may end up reading at only a seventh or eighth grade level. Health literacy also includes numeracy skills. For example, understanding probability and risk, calculating blood sugar levels, measuring medications, and understanding nutrition labels all require math skills.

In addition to basic literacy skills, health literacy requires knowledge of health and medical issues. People with limited health literacy often lack the knowledge or even are misinformed about the human body as well as the nature and cause of disease. As such, they may not understand the relationship between lifestyle factors such as diet and exercise and various health outcomes. Furthermore, their ability to engage in self-care and chronic disease management may be impaired.

It has been estimated that only 12% of adults have proficient health literacy. In other words, nearly 9 of 10 adults may lack the skills necessary to properly manage their health and prevent disease. Populations that frequently experience low health literacy include older people, racial and ethnic minorities, people without a high school diploma or GED, individuals with low incomes, non-native speakers of English, and people with chronic disease.

Why is the health literacy of your patients important to you in your role as a healthcare professional? Those individuals with low health literacy are more likely to:

- Overlook important preventative measures such as mammograms, Pap smears, colonoscopies, prostate examinations, and flu shots.
- Have a chronic disease, be less able to manage their care effectively, and be less likely to get the health care they need.
- Enter the healthcare system when they are sicker.
- Go to the emergency room and be hospitalized.
- Lack health insurance.
- Have a sense of shame regarding their lack of skills and may hide their difficulties to maintain their dignity.
- Be noncompliant with doctor's instructions and make medication errors.
- Have poorer health outcomes and higher healthcare costs.

The HCP may employ a variety of strategies to communicate and interact most effectively with patients with low health literacy, including the following:

1 *Evaluate the patient's understanding before, during, and after the introduction of information or instruction.* Ask the patient to explain the information back to you in their own words or to demonstrate the skills that you have taught them.
2 *Limit the number of messages given to a patient at any one time.* Less than half of the information provided to patients during each visit is retained.
3 *Use "plain language."* Plain language is communication that the patient can understand the first time they hear it or read it. This method of communication is characterized by the following:
   - Information that is organized so that the most important points are delivered first;
   - Information that is broken down into understandable chunks;
   - Language that is simple with clearly defined medical terminology;
   - The use of the active voice.

Remain mindful that language that may be plain to one patient or group of patients may not be plain to others. Know your audience! For example, older adults may respond to certain kinds of language differently from younger adults. This may also be the case for different cultural or ethnic groups.

   4 *Supplement instructions with pictures.* Simple line drawings may help patients understand complicated or abstract medical concepts. Images must be placed in context. In other words, when illustrating internal body parts, include an outline of the outside of the body.

   5 *Tailor medication schedules to fit a patient's daily routine.* Daily events (e.g., meals) or tasks (e.g., brushing teeth) that serve as reminders may improve patient compliance.

   6 *Prepare written forms of communication at a fifth- to sixth-grade reading level and in a format that appears easy to read.* This reading level will reach the majority of patients and is recommended for all health education materials. Use at least 12-point font. Avoid using all capital letters, italics, or ornate script. Use headings and bullets to break up the text. Include spaces between sections and maintain wide margins around the text.

   7 *Provide or serve as a reader for forms or written information.* A family member may also fill this role and will be available to continue to assist the patient at home.

Language Barriers

When the patient and the HCP do not speak the same language, the opportunity to develop rapport is reduced. In this case, the use of "small talk" to obtain relevant clinical information from the patient and to emotionally engage with the patient is limited. Instead of communicating directly with each other, the patient and the HCP must rely on a medical interpreter to deliver their messages. Furthermore, when the patient and the HCP do not understand each other's language, not only may the patient be less likely to effectively convey their complaints and concerns, but the HCP may also be less likely to effectively convey their diagnosis and recommendations. Recent studies show that a language barrier between a healthcare provider and a pediatric patient and their family can cause an increased use of diagnostic tests in an emergency department as well as increased rates of hospitalizations. Adverse medical events in these hospitalized patients are also more common. Therefore, it should be evident that the effective use of a qualified medical interpreter is of paramount importance. Specifically, the use of nonprofessional interpreters should be avoided. There are significant disadvantages to the use of friends or family members as medical interpreters. These individuals are often unfamiliar with complex medical information.

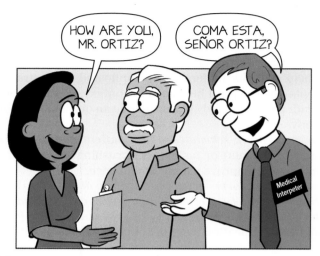

FIGURE 6-1. **Language Barriers.** When the patient and the HCP do not speak the same language, they must rely on a medical interpreter to deliver their messages.

As a result, nonprofessional interpreters are far more likely to incorrectly translate words and phases from the HCP to the patient. A second disadvantage involves the loss of patient confidentiality. The patient may not feel comfortable being candid in the presence of children, parents, or friends. Consequently, they may withhold potentially important details of their condition.

The HCP may employ a variety of strategies to work more effectively with a medical interpreter, including the following:

1 *Look at and speak directly to the patient.* To facilitate more direct interaction between the patient and the HCP, the interpreter should

TABLE 6-1

Summary of Strategies for Communicating with Patients Through a Medical Interpreter

- Look at and speak directly to the patient
- Use short sentences
- Avoid the use of informal and unprofessional vocabulary
- Remain patient and understanding
- Observe the patient's nonverbal messages
- Repeat important information
- Ask the patient to repeat important instructions or information in their own words
- Avoid the use of ad hoc interpreters

stand behind and a little to the side of the patient. This will enable the HCP to avoid addressing the interpreter ("Tell Mrs. Martinez. . . ." or "Ask Mr. Ngyuen. . . .") Instead, the HCP will be better able to address the patient directly ("I am prescribing blood pressure medication for you, Mrs. Martinez" or "Can you tell me exactly where the pain is, Mr. Nguyen?")

2 *Use short sentences.* The use of long, involved sentences and paragraphs would tend to increase the likelihood of error during interpreting.

3 *Avoid the use of informal and unprofessional vocabulary.* This would include slang, similes, metaphors, and figures of speech. Instead, use formal but simple speech and vocabulary.

Example: "That new doctor *rocks*."
Better: "That new doctor is *excellent*."

Example: "He is as *healthy as a horse*." or "She is *sick as a dog*."
Better: "He is *very healthy*." or "She is *quite sick*."

Example: "Have you been feeling *blue* lately?"
Better: "Have you been feeling *sad*?"

Example: "Don't worry that the medication was not effective. There is more than one way to *skin a cat*."
Better: "Don't worry that the medication was not effective. There are *other options for your treatment*."

4 *Remain patient and understanding.* Interaction with a patient through an interpreter takes more time. Not all words exist in all languages. Therefore, the interpreter may be required to use many words to express the same meaning as a single word or phrase. In addition, the interpreter may occasionally need to pause to ask the HCP for further explanation or clarification in order to most accurately interpret the message.

5 *Observe the patient's nonverbal messages.* As discussed in Chapter 2, the patient may convey a great deal of information nonverbally. This may help to clarify the patient's feelings and, perhaps, their message.

6 *Repeat important information.* As will be discussed in Chapter 7, "Patient Education," repetition of the information serves to reinforce the message. This will also provide additional opportunities for the patient to ask questions regarding this critical information.

ROLE **PLAY** **Language Barriers**
With a partner, identify other instances where there may be a formal and an informal way to convey a message in a clinical setting. For each pair of messages, discuss how a patient for whom English is not their first language may misunderstand the informal message.

FIGURE 6-2. Visual Impairment. Except for their vision loss, visually impaired patients are normal and should be treated as such.

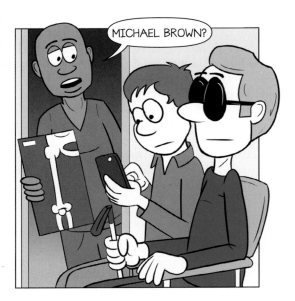

MICHAEL BROWN?

7 *Employ "teach back."* In other words, ask the patient to repeat important instructions or information in their own words. This will confirm that the patient has accurately interpreted and understood the message conveyed by the HCP.

Visual Impairment

Vision loss refers to difficulty seeing, even when wearing corrective lenses (glasses or contacts), as well as complete blindness. This is a substantial problem in the United States since well over 25 million Americans report experiencing significant vision loss. However, except for their visual impairment, these patients are normal and they should be treated as such. As with language barriers, visual impairment does not have to lead to impaired communication.

The HCP may employ a variety of strategies to communicate and interact most effectively with patients who are visually impaired. These strategies, which are based primarily on courtesy, respect, and common sense, include the following:

1 *Greet the patient.* As you approach the patient or enter the clinical area, greet the patient, clearly identify who you are, and speak in a normal tone of voice. Shake hands with the patient but only if they offer their hand.
2 *Speak directly to the patient.* During your conversation (i.e., face-to-face), speak directly to the patient and use their name so that

TABLE 6-2

Summary of Strategies for Communicating with Patients Who Are Visually Impaired

- Greet the patient
- Shake hands with the patient only if they offer their hand
- Speak directly to the patient
- Tell the patient that you will be touching them before you do so
- Explain to the patient what you are doing as you are doing it
- Be verbally descriptive
- Use the words "look" and "see" normally
- Tell the patient when you are leaving the area
- Do not attempt to guide the patient without first asking
- Never touch or distract the patient's service dog
- Walk with the patient between you and the service dog
- Be patient, considerate, and take your time
- Provide reasonable accommodations

they know that you are addressing them. Adopt a normal position (i.e., sitting or standing as appropriate). If there are other individuals involved in the conversation, such as family members or other HCPs, specify whom you are addressing.

3 *Tell the patient that you will be touching them before you do so.* Never surprise a visually impaired patient with needles, a cold stethoscope, or other medical objects and devices. As with all patients, explain what you are doing as you are doing it.

4 *Be verbally descriptive.* When providing instructions, be descriptive when conveying information that would be visually obvious to patients with normal vision. Do not point or gesture as this is of little or no value to these patients.

5 *Use the words "look" and "see" normally.* Visually impaired patients have the same vocabulary as sighted people and these words are a natural part of conversation. Avoiding them may create an awkward or uncomfortable situation.

6 *Tell the patient when you are leaving the area.* Let the patient know if other individuals will remain in the area or if the patient will be alone. Similarly, inform the patient when you return.

7 *Do not attempt to guide the patient without first asking.* If assistance is welcome, allow the patient to take your arm above the elbow or to place their hand on your shoulder in order to control their own movements.

8 *Never touch or distract the patient's service dog.* When a service dog is wearing its harness, it is "working" and should not be touched or

Interacting with a Visually Impaired Patient

In groups of three to four—one blind patient, one HCP, and one to two observers—take turns playing the patient and the HCP and acting out the following scenarios.

1 A medical assistant greets the patient in the waiting room, takes the patient to the examination room, and then leaves.
2 A nurse enters the room and takes the pulse of the patient at their right wrist. The nurse then obtains the patient's weight.
3 A radiology technologist instructs the patient to position their left arm in the prone position followed by the supine position for x-rays.

Following each role play scenario, discuss the interaction between the patient and the HCP. What was effective in facilitating the interaction? What had a negative impact on the interaction? How did any inappropriate behaviors on the part of the HCP make the patient feel?

distracted by anyone but the dog's companion. If the patient's service dog is resting, ask for the patient's permission before touching the dog.

9 *Walk with the patient between you and the service dog.* If a patient with a service dog needs additional assistance from you, approach and walk on the other side of the patient. In other words, walk with

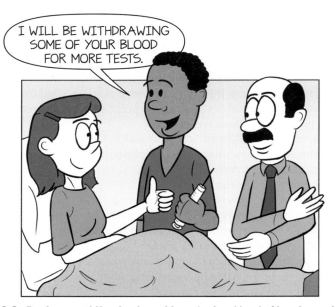

FIGURE 6-3. Deafness and Hearing Loss. Many deaf and hard of hearing patients are good speech readers. Many others prefer communicating via American Sign Language (ASL). Therefore, it may be necessary to use a professional ASL interpreter in the clinical setting.

the patient between you and the dog. The service dog has been trained to understand that he is still in charge and is responsible for his companion.

10 *Provide reasonable accommodations.* Patients who are essentially or totally blind may require medical information that is prepared in audiotape, or Braille formats. Patients who have low vision may require written materials that are printed with 14-, 16- or 18-point font, with margins that are at least one inch on all sides, with at least 1½ spaces between the lines of type, and with significant contrast between the print and the background (i.e., black print on white paper).

Deafness and Hearing Loss

The term "deaf" refers to those patients who are unable to hear well enough to rely on their hearing and use it as a means of processing information. (The lower case *deaf* is used when referring to the audiologic

TABLE 6-3

Summary of Strategies for Communicating with Patients Who Are Deaf or Hard of Hearing

- Interact directly with the patient
- Record and respect the patient's preferred method of communication
- Position yourself in front of the patient
- Be sure that the patient sees you approach
- Gain the patient's attention before you speak
- Speak clearly, in a normal tone of voice, a little more loudly, and at a moderate pace
- Pause between phrases
- Avoid having anything in your mouth
- Optimize conditions for speech reading
- Minimize the use of medical terminology
- Maintain eye contact with the patient
- Use short, simple sentences
- Include the use of nonverbal communication
- Observe the patient's nonverbal behavior
- Do not talk over your shoulder or from an unobservable area
- Minimize any background noise as much as possible
- Rephrase the message
- Write the message
- Use a professional interpreter
- Indicate a change in topic
- Supplement the conversation with visual aids
- Ask the patient to repeat the information
- Be patient and considerate

condition. The uppercase *Deaf* is used when referring to a particular group of deaf individuals who share a language, American Sign Language, and a culture.) The term "hard of hearing" refers to those patients who have some hearing and are able to use it for communication purposes. These patients are described as having mild to moderate hearing loss.

As with vision loss, hearing loss is also a substantial problem in the United States. More than 28 million Americans are deaf or hard of hearing. Because the majority of these individuals are 65 years of age and older, the number of deaf and hard of hearing patients is expected to increase substantially in the coming years as the population ages. Therefore, HCPs must learn how to communicate effectively with this growing patient population. Similar to those patients with vision loss, patients who are deaf or hard of hearing are normal and should be treated as such.

Ineffective communication between the HCP and deaf or hard of hearing patients can lead to misdiagnosis and medication errors, as well as potential patient embarrassment, anxiety or fear. The Americans with Disabilities Act (ADA) requires clinicians to provide auxiliary or supplemental protocols so they may effectively communicate with deaf and hard of hearing patients as well as deaf and hard of hearing family members. For example, it may be necessary to use a professional interpreter of American Sign Language (ASL) in the clinical setting. Patients who were born bilaterally deaf are likely to communicate by way of ASL, which is not based on English and uses a different sentence structure and grammar. Furthermore, only about 30% of English sounds are visible on the lips, which may make speech reading difficult. In fact, there are instances when an interpreter may become essential in facilitating the communication between the HCP and the patient. For example, the topic of the communication may be critically important, such as the details of a complex surgical procedure, or time constraints may leave no room for slow or ponderous communication. As in the case with the use of a medical interpreter, if the patient uses a sign language interpreter, speak directly to the patient and not the interpreter.

The HCP must remember to be patient and considerate. Remain mindful that everyone, especially hard of hearing patients, will hear and understand less well when they are tired, ill, or in pain. It can be a marked strain for these patients when they have to remain attentive for long periods of time. If at some point the patient does not understand you, ***never*** say "It's not important," as this is dismissive and disrespectful to the patient.

The HCP may employ a variety of strategies to communicate and interact most effectively with patients who are deaf or hard of hearing. As with those suggested for patients with visual impairment, these strategies are based on courtesy, respect, and common sense.

1 *Be sure that the patient sees you approach.* This will help to avoid startling them.

2 *Interact directly with the patient.* Focus on your patient as opposed to friends or family members who may have accompanied them. This patient has lost their ability to hear, not their individuality, dignity, or intellectual competence. In addition, you must be positioned in front of the patient. If possible, be at the same level as they are. Look directly at the patient. Avoid speaking to them while reviewing or writing in their medical record or otherwise multitasking. Finally, minimize any background noise as much as possible. Most hard of hearing individuals have greater difficulty understanding speech when there is extraneous or competing noise.

3 *Record and respect the patient's preferred method of communication.*

4 *If your patient hears better in one ear than the other, make note of this in the patient's medical record and position yourself accordingly.*

5 *Gain the patient's attention before you speak.* Say the patient's name or make a small gesture such as raising your hand or touching the patient's arm. This will enable the patient to focus their attention and avoid missing words at the beginning of the conversation. Remain mindful of any special situations where a hard of hearing patient may be required to turn off their hearing aid because of equipment interference. In these instances, the HCP must make a point of gaining the patient's attention or explaining what is required of them during the procedure.

6 *Speak clearly, in a normal tone of voice, a little more loudly, and at a moderate pace. Pause between phrases.* Do not shout or exaggerate your mouth movements. Shouting will distort the sounds of speech and may make speech reading more difficult. In addition, loud speech may be painful to a patient wearing a hearing aid and will have no added benefit for the profoundly deaf patient. Finally, shouting may result in the loss of privacy for the patient. Pausing between phrases will provide the patient with time to process what you have said.

7 *Optimize conditions for speech reading.* Many deaf and hard of hearing patients will be good speech readers. Ensure that the light is behind the patient and does not shine in their eyes. With the light behind them, they will see your face and lips clearly. Avoid having obstacles in front of your face such as your hands or a surgical mask as this will obscure your face and lips. In addition, avoid having anything in your mouth. Items such as gum, candy, and pens will make your speech more difficult to understand. Do not talk over your shoulder or from an unobservable area. For example, a radiology technologist will typically say "hold your breath" from behind a protective screen. An alternative approach is the use of a light as a signal for required actions.

8 *Minimize the use of medical terminology.* The HCP must remain mindful that medical terminology may pose a special problem for deaf and hard of hearing patients. Speech readers typically rely on previous experience with vocabulary and various topics. An overwhelming amount of new medical vocabulary may make it difficult for the patient to follow and understand the HCP.

9 *Maintain eye contact with the patient.* The patient is likely to follow your glance around the room, expecting that someone has entered or that something is happening in another part of the room. Alternatively, the patient may misinterpret your random eye movements as disinterest or discomfort with them.

10 *Include the use and observation of nonverbal communication.* When appropriate, use nonverbal forms of communication such as facial expressions and gestures to supplement your verbal message. In addition, observe the patient's nonverbal behavior. If there is any sign of confusion, hurt, or misunderstanding, immediately and tactfully ask the patient if they have understood you. You may also ask leading questions of the patient in order to determine whether your message was accurately interpreted.

11 *Rephrase or write the message.* If the patient has difficulty understanding your message, find a different way of saying the same thing. Do not repeat the same words over and over. For example, if the patient did not understand when you said, "This injection could sting," repeat it once. If this is not successful, then reword your sentence to "This shot may hurt." If rephrasing the message does not work, write some of or the entire message for the patient. Write legibly! The benefit of writing, however, may be limited. Writing is slow and cumbersome. In addition, patients with limited verbal skills may have some difficulty expressing themselves using a written format.

12 *Indicate a change in topic.* When changing the subject during a conversation, be sure that the patient is aware of what the new subject is. Sudden shifts in topic can be very confusing and may lead to a breakdown in effective communication.

13 *Supplement the conversation with visual aids.* The use of visual aids may significantly enhance the effectiveness of the communication. Any visual aids should be in an upright position and as close to you as possible without blocking your face. This will allow the patient to observe you and the visual aid simultaneously and avoid having to look back and forth between you and the object. Consider the meteorologist, or weatherman, on television. They are able to gesture toward the weather map behind them while speaking directly to the camera. With practice, an HCP may also be able to gesture toward a visual aid while speaking directly to the patient without constantly changing position or looking away from the patient.

14 *Employ teach back.* As with the patient who speaks another language, ask the patient to repeat the information. When providing the hard of hearing patient with specific information such as an appointment time or details regarding a medication (e.g., dosages, how many times per day to take it), have the patient repeat the specifics back to you. Many numbers and words sound alike.

Advanced Age

The size of the elderly population in the United States is increasing markedly. When American soldiers returned home after World War II, the United States experienced a profound and prolonged surge in the birth rate. Individuals who were born between 1946 and 1964 are now referred to as "Baby Boomers." In 2010, there were an estimated 76 million Baby Boomers. The first of these turned 60 years old in 2006. As this group continues to age, the nature of the overall American population will change dramatically. The U.S. Census Bureau has estimated that by the year 2030, more than 58 million Americans will be age 65 or older.

Declining health and complex disease management in the elderly results in multiple visits to doctors and other healthcare providers

---

ROLE PLAY **Communicating with a Deaf Patient**

In groups of three to four—one deaf patient, one HCP, and one to two observers—take turns playing the patient and the HCP and recording the following portion of the patient's medical history (see Fig. 5-2):

1 **Do you wear corrective lenses?**
2 **Do you have frequent or severe headaches?**
3 **Have you had tuberculosis?**
4 **Do you have hay fever or allergic rhinitis?**
5 **Do you have asthma?**
6 **Do you have any pain or pressure in your chest?**
7 **Have you had any broken bones?**
8 **Do you have frequent indigestion?**
9 **Do you have trouble sleeping?**
10 **Have you had chemotherapy?**
11 **Are you depressed or excessively worried?**
12 **Do you use tobacco?**

Discuss what strategies and techniques were effective in facilitating communication with the patient. What impaired communication? How did any inappropriate behaviors on the part of the HCP make the patient feel?

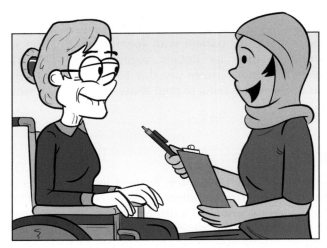

FIGURE 6-4. Advanced Age. Communication between elderly patients and their HCPs may be impaired by several factors including vision and hearing loss, decline in memory, and the slower processing of information.

each year. Unfortunately, communication between these older patients and their HCPs may be impaired by several factors including sensory loss (e.g., vision loss and hearing loss as discussed previously in this chapter), decline in memory, and the slower processing of information. As such, healthcare providers must adapt their communication in order to remain most effective with their older patients.

The HCP may employ a variety of strategies to communicate and interact most effectively with patients of advanced age, including the following:

1 *Schedule older patients earlier in the day and allot extra time.* The elderly tend to become tired later in the day. Furthermore, an early appointment will allow you to spend extra time with these patients as you are more likely to be running on time. Due to their declining health, more medical information may need to be conveyed to these patients. As mentioned previously, some of these patients may process this information more slowly than younger patients. Both of these factors may require the HCP to spend more time with their elderly patients.

2 *Speak slowly, clearly, and loudly.* A slower pace will allow the patient to process the information conveyed to them and commit it to memory. In addition, it is best to use simple words and short sentences. Choose words that are familiar to the patient. Simplified instructions will be easier for the patient to follow.

TABLE 6-4

Summary of Strategies for Communicating with Patients of Advanced Age

- Schedule older patients earlier in the day
- Allot extra time
- Speak slowly, clearly and loudly
- Use simple words and short sentences
- Repeat important information
- Write down the instructions
- Focus on one topic at a time
- Minimize distractions
- Face the patient and maintain eye contact
- Use visual aids
- Provide an opportunity for patients to ask questions

3 *Repeat important information and write down instructions.* Frequently repeat and summarize important information for the patient. Written instructions provide a reference for the patient should they forget the information when they leave the medical office or clinic.

4 *Focus on one topic at a time and minimize distractions.* This will reduce the likelihood of confusion on the part of the patient.

5 *Face the patient and maintain eye contact.* Sitting face-to-face will facilitate communication with those patients who experience vision loss or hearing loss. It will also help to minimize distractions for these patients and allow them to focus on the HCP.

6 *Use visual aids.* Charts, models, and figures will supplement your verbal message and aid visual learners. As with other patients, provide an opportunity for patients to ask questions. This will confirm their understanding of the information.

Delirium and Dementia

In addition to a decline in their physical health, some elderly patients also have a decline in their cognitive abilities. In other words, they are more likely to experience confusion. There are two types of confusion. *Acute confusion,* also referred to as *delirium,* occurs when a patient undergoes a temporary or reversible period of disorientation, hallucinations, or delusions. During these episodes, the patient will find it difficult to focus attention and to rest or sleep. Acute confusion typically has an abrupt onset, which is associated with a specific risk factor or cause. For example, elderly patients often metabolize gen-

Use of Visual Aids
With a partner—one elderly patient and one HCP—take turns playing the patient and the HCP and acting out each of the following scenarios.

1 Using a skeleton, a radiology technologist indicates to the patient the location of their ruptured intervertebral disc.
2 Using an anatomic chart, a nurse describes where gastroesophageal reflux takes place and why it feels like "heartburn."
3 Using an anatomic chart, a medical assistant indicates which muscle the patient strained while lifting a heavy box.

Discuss what was effective in facilitating communication with the patient. What impaired communication?

eral anesthesia differently from younger patients, which may result in profound delirium for a period of time. Episodes may last for hours or days. *Chronic confusion,* also referred to as *dementia,* occurs when a patient undergoes a progressive, irreversible decline in mental function, characterized by memory impairment, deficits in reasoning,

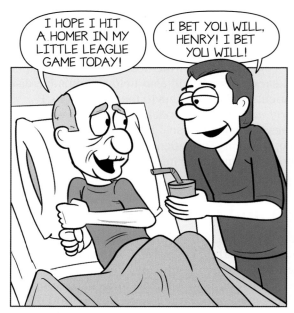

FIGURE 6-5. Dementia. Chronic confusion, or dementia, is characterized by a progressive, irreversible decline in mental function and includes memory impairment as well as deficits in reasoning, judgment, abstract thought, comprehension, and learning.

judgment, abstract thought, comprehension, learning, task execution, and use of language. Chronic confusion, which may involve degenerative processes, typically has an insidious onset that occurs over months or years.

The aging of the population has been accompanied by a marked increase in the prevalence of dementia in the United States. Approximately 10% of patients older than 65, and almost half of patients older than age 85, have some form of dementia. The most common of these is Alzheimer's disease, which accounts for 65% of dementia cases. The Alzheimer's Association reports that as many as 5 million Americans have this disease and more than twice that number will be afflicted in the next 30 years.

Effectively communicating with cognitively impaired patients, especially those with dementia, is particularly challenging for healthcare providers. The HCP may employ a variety of strategies to communicate and interact most effectively with these patients including the following:

1 *Expect an increase in confusion from the patient upon waking up as well as when "sundowning."* Many patients with dementia experience heightened confusion later in the day, hence, the term "sundowning."
2 *Approach the patient from the front and call the patient by name.* The patient may be startled if they are touched unexpectedly or if they are approached from behind.
3 *Respect the patient's personal space and observe their reaction as you move closer.* Begin by positioning yourself about an arm's length from the patient.

TABLE 6-5

Summary of Strategies for Communicating with Patients with Delirium or Dementia

- Expect an increase in confusion when the patient wakes up as well as "sundowning"
- Approach the patient from the front and call the patient by name
- Respect the patient's personal space and observe their reaction as you move closer
- Avoid sudden movements that may startle or irritate the patient
- Speak slowly and distinctly in a low-pitched voice
- Ask one question at a time
- Give one step directions and instruction
- Remain mindful of your nonverbal messages
- Do not disagree or argue with the patient

4 *Avoid sudden movements that may startle or irritate the patient.* Maintain a friendly facial expression. Be calm and reassuring. Exhibit interest and maintain eye contact. Remain mindful that these patients may be coping with anxiety, loss of self-esteem, irritability, or depression.

5 *Speak slowly and distinctly in a low-pitched voice.* Use simple words and sentences. Be precise. Avoid expressions that may be ambiguous or confusing. For example, say, "Your hat is on the table," instead of "Here you go."

6 *Ask one question at a time.* This will help to minimize confusion. Allow adequate time for the patient to respond. If the patient has difficulty understanding the question, uses the wrong word, or cannot identify the correct word for their reply, rephrase your question in the form of a statement that may provide the patient's desired response.

7 *Give one-step directions and instructions.* Too many steps at one time or many directions too quickly will overwhelm the patient and result in confusion. Allow adequate time for the patient to perform the activity.

8 *Remain mindful of your nonverbal messages.* Patients with dementia may be particularly perceptive to your body language and mood. Use nonverbal communication to send calming messages to the patient. For example, smile and nod at the patient. Nonverbal gestures and pointing may also be used to supplement your verbal message.

9 *Do not disagree or argue with the patient.* Patients with dementia may have delusions or hallucinations. Respond to the emotion conveyed by their story. Remain soothing and supportive of these patients.

ROLE **PLAY**   **Interacting with a Patient with Dementia**
In groups of three to four—one patient, one patient care technician (PCT), and one to two observers—act out the following scenario.

An 87-year-old man lives in a nursing home. Over the last several months he has become increasingly confused, especially upon waking in the morning as well as in the evening. A PCT comes to get the man ready for dinner. The PCT is to help him comb his hair and put on his bathrobe. During their interaction, the man asks when his mother will return from the grocery store. He is worried that his dog, Max, is getting hungry.

Discuss what was effective in facilitating the interaction with the patient. What had a negative impact on this interaction? How did any inappropriate behaviors on the part of the PCT affect the patient?

REVIEW QUESTIONS

OBJECTIVE QUESTIONS

1 Nine out of ten adults have proficient health literacy. *(True or false?)*
2 Individuals with low health literacy have poorer health outcomes and higher healthcare costs. *(True or false?)*
3 Family members are preferred as medical interpreters for patients who speak another language because they know the patient well. *(True or false?)*
4 It is best to never touch or pet a blind patient's service dog without first asking. *(True or false?)*
5 Shouting will distort the sounds of speech and make speech reading more difficult. *(True or false?)*
6 It is better to schedule elderly patients later in the day as they are more alert at this time. *(True or false?)*
7 Visual aids are useful in supplementing your communication with most of your patients. *(True or false?)*
8 Acute confusion is referred to as dementia. *(True or false?)*
9 It is recommended that delusional patients are corrected and informed about what is really happening. *(True or false?)*

SHORT ANSWER QUESTIONS

1 Discuss at least three strategies that will facilitate communication with a patient with low health literacy. Explain why these strategies are helpful.
2 Discuss at least three strategies that will facilitate communication with a patient who speaks another language. Explain why these strategies are helpful.
3 Discuss at least three strategies that will facilitate communication with a patient who is blind or visually impaired. Explain why these strategies are helpful.
4 Discuss at least three strategies that will facilitate communication with a patient who is deaf or hard of hearing. Explain why these strategies are helpful.
5 Discuss at least three strategies that will facilitate communication with a patient who is elderly. Explain why these strategies are helpful.
6 Distinguish between delirium and dementia.
7 Discuss at least three strategies that will facilitate communication with a patient with dementia. Explain why these strategies are helpful.

CLINICAL APPLICATIONS

1 Watch an episode of your favorite medical drama while facing away from the television. Keeping in mind that you cannot see the health-care provider, assume the role of the patient in the episode. Discuss the interaction between you as the patient and the provider. Are you able to completely understand all of the provider's messages? What nonverbal messages do you believe you are missing by not actually seeing the provider? If, indeed, the provider were interacting with a blind patient, what changes would you recommend that would improve communication and make the patient more comfortable during the encounter?

2 A radiology technologist in mammography must perform a mammogram on a deaf patient. Discuss the behaviors that may be employed to interact with and instruct the patient during the procedure.

3 Design a one-page brochure regarding a disease that occurs frequently in the elderly (e.g., heart disease, osteoporosis). Include the symptoms and the treatment options. Prepare this brochure with the assumption that the patient will have some degree of vision loss. Identify the qualities of your brochure that make it suitable for this particular patient.

4 A nurse must wake up a 92-year-old female patient at 2 a.m. in order to listen to her chest for signs of congestion and to administer her medication in the form of a capsule. Discuss the behaviors that may be employed to complete these tasks while calming and reassuring the patient.

Fundamental Writing Skills

The section in the writing skills chapter you should complete at the end of Chapter 6 is Section 10-6. You can find this section on pages 226–230.

SUGGESTED FURTHER READING

1. Alzbrain.org. Communication tips when interacting with dementia patients. Retrieved April 2010 from www.alzbrain.org/pdf/handouts/2059.%20communicATION%20TIPS20FOR%20DEMENTIA%20PATIENTS.

2. American Foundation for the Blind. Facts and figures on Americans with vision loss. Retrieved April 2010 from http://www.afb.org/Section.asp?SectionID=15&TopicID=413&DocumentID=4900.

3. Baby Boomer Headquarters. The boomer stats. Retrieved April 2010 from http://www.bbhq.com/bomrstat.htm.

4. Breen LM. What should I do if my patient does not speak English? *JAMA*. 1999;282:819.

5. Brown WS. Communicating with hearing-impaired patients, *West J Med*. 1977; 127(2):164–168.

6. Center for Health Care Strategies. Health Literacy Fact Sheets. Retrieved April 2010 from www.chcs.org/publications3960/publications_show.htm?doc_id=291711.

7. Centers for Disease Control and Prevention, Division of Health Communication and Marketing. What we know about health literacy. Retrieved April 2010 from http://www.cdc.gov/healthmarketing/resources.htm.

8. Chen A. Doctoring across the language divide. *Health Affairs*. 2006; 25(3): 808–813.

9. Cohen AL, Rivara F, Marcuse EK, et al. Are language barriers associated with serious medical events in hospitalized pediatric patients? *Pediatrics*. 2005; 116(3):575–579.

10. ElderCare Online. Communicating with impaired elderly persons. Retrieved April 2010 from http://www.ec-online.net/Knowledge/Articles/communication.html.

11. Glassman P. Health literacy. http://nnlm.gov/outreach/consumer/hlthlit.html.

12. Gregg J, Saha S. Communicative competence: a framework for understanding language barriers in health care. *J Gen Intern Med*. 2007; 22 (Suppl 2):368–370.

13. Hearing Loss Web. Tips for the hearing person. Retrieved April 2010 from http://www.hearinglossweb.com/Issues/OralCommunications/tips1.htm.

14. Hampers LC, Cha S, Gutglass DJ, et al. Language barriers and resource utilization in a pediatric emergency department. *Pediatrics*. 1999; 103: 1253–1256.

15. Hampers LC, McNulty JE. Professional interpreters and bilingual physicians in a pediatric emergency department: effect on resource utilization. *Arch Pediatr Adolesce Med*. 2002;156:1108–1113.

16. Hilgers J. Comforting a confused patient. *Nursing*. 2003;33(1):48–50.

17. Iezzoni LI, O'Day BL, Killeen M, et al. Communicating about health care: observations from persons who are deaf or hard of hearing, *Ann Intern Med*. 2004;140:356–362.

18. Kallail KJ. Communicating with patients at risk for low health literacy. *Kans J Med*. 2007, 22–26.

19. Kelly CK. Learning to communicate with *all* your patients, hiring interpreters—and other tips—to work with patients who are deaf or don't speak English, *Amer Coll Phys Observer*. November, 1997. Retrieved April 2010 from http://www.acpinternist.org/archives/1997/11/learn-com.htm.

20. Kricos PB. Communication strategies: it takes two to tango!—part one. Retrieved April 2010 from http://www.hearinglossweb.com/Issues/Oral Communications/Strategies/strat.htm.

21. Kricos PB. Communication strategies: it takes two to tango!—part two. Retrieved April 2010 from http://www.hearinglossweb.com/Issues/Oral Communications/Strategies/stratb.htm.

22. National Association of the Deaf. Community and culture—Frequently asked questions. Retrieved April 2010 from http://www.nad.org/issues/american-sign-language/community-and-culture-faq.

23. National Association of the Deaf. Resource Summary Page. Retrieved April 2010 from http://www.icdri.org/dhhi/national_association_of_the_deaf.htm.

24. Osborne H. In other words . . . when vision is an issue . . . communicating with patients who are visually impaired. Retrieved April 2010 from http://www.healthliteracy.com/article.asp?PageID=3774.

25. Parker SO. Increasing physician-patient communication in the elderly. *HealthMad.* September 2008. Retrieved April 2010 from http://www.healthmad.com/Senior-Health/Increasing-Physician-Patient-Communication-in-the- Elderly.254003.

26. Partida Y. Language barriers and the patient encounter. *Virtual Mentor.* 2007;9(8):566–571. Retrieved April 2010 from http://virtualmentor.ama-assn.org/2007/08/msoc1-0708.html.

27. Quick Guide to Health Literacy. Health literacy basics. Retrieved April 2010 from http://www.health.gov/communication/literacy/quickguide/factsbasic.htm.

28. Quick Guide to Health Literacy. Health literacy and health outcomes. Retrieved April 2010 from http://www.health.gov/communication/literacy/quickguide/factsliteracy.htm.

29. Quick Guide to Health Literacy. Improve the usability of health information. Retrieved April 2010 from http://www.health.gov/communication/literacy/quickguide/healthinfo.htm.

30. Quick Guide to Health Literacy. Improve the usability of health services. Retrieved April 2010 from http://www.health.gov/communication/literacy/quickguide/services.htm.

31. Quick Guide to Health Literacy. Advocate for health literacy in your organization. Retrieved April 2010 from http://www.health.gov/communication/literacy/quickguide/advocate.htm.

32. Raynor DK, Yerassimou N. Medicines information—leaving blind people behind? *Br J Med.* 1997;315:268.

33. Robinson TE, White GL, Houchins JC. Improving communication with older patients: tips from the literature. American Academy of Family Physicians. *Fam Pract Manage.* September 2006. Retrieved April 2010 from http://www.aafp.org/fpm/2006/0900/p73.html.

34. Shank SL, Ratchford J. Confused about confusion? *National Center of Continuing Education.* Retrieved April 2010 from http://www.nursece.com/onlinecourses/3178.html.

35. Stevens S. Assisting the blind and visually impaired: guidelines for eye health workers and other helpers. *Commun Eye Health.* 2003;16(45):7–9.

36. *Taber's Cyclopedia Medical Dictionary,* 20th ed. Philadelphia: F. A. Davis Co; 2005.

37. University of Michigan Medical School. Cultural Competence for Clinicians, How to work with a foreign language interpreter. Retrieved April 2010 from http://www.med.umich.edu/pteducation/cultcomp.htm.

38. U.S. Census Bureau. Oldest baby boomers turn 60! Retrieved April 2010 from http://www.census.gov/Press-Release/www/releases/archives/facts_for_features_special_editions/006105.html.

39. U.S. Department of Labor, Office of Disability Employment Policy. Communicating with and about people with disabilities. Retrieved April 2010 from http://www.dol.gov/odep/pubs/fact/comucate.htm.
40. Wagenaar DB. Communicating with the elderly. *Dial and Diag.* April, 2007. Retrieved April 2010 from https://www.do-online.org/pdf/pub_dd0407wagenaar.pdf.

7

PATIENT EDUCATION

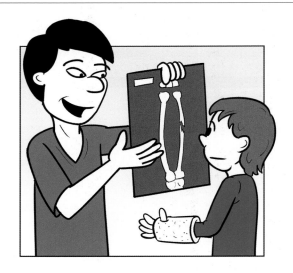

OBJECTIVES

- Identify the benefits of patient education
- Describe the factors that determine the type of instruction needed
- Describe the factors that may influence the patient's response to the instruction
- Design behavioral objectives, determine the content that should be included, and discuss the factors that contribute to clear communication during a teaching session
- Distinguish the three types of learning styles
- Explain how interaction and two-way communication with the patient enhances the educational process
- Discuss the strategies that contribute to effective patient instruction
- Describe the benefits and identify the potential limitations of using visual aids and written materials

Introduction

Benefits of Patient Education

Healthcare professionals (HCPs) are knowledgeable about health, disease, diagnostic procedures, and treatment regimens, particularly in their areas of specialization. However, most patients are not well informed or familiar with these issues. This lack of knowledge may prevent patients from making good decisions about their health and, therefore, may have a negative impact on their health status. In addition to giving care to a patient, another important service that HCPs may provide as part of their practice is patient education. There are three important objectives of patient education that may result in positive health outcomes:

- Changing health behaviors
- Improving health status
- Improving patient compliance

An important goal of patient education is to change the health behaviors of patients. For example, the HCP may instruct a patient on the proper use of contraceptives, good nutrition, the detrimental effects of smoking and drinking, or the beneficial effects of regular exercise. This education may encourage patients to take an active role in their health and medical care. In fact, evidence suggests that when patients are confident that they can positively influence their health, they are more likely to do so than those patients who do not have that confidence.

A second goal is to improve the health status of patients. For example, instruction about the use of sunscreen may decrease the risk of a patient developing melanoma. Instruction regarding the performance of routine breast examinations may result in the early detection of breast cancer and, therefore, a markedly improved prognosis for the patient.

Finally, patient education may result in better compliance with treatment programs. For example, patients with hypertension often have no outward symptoms even though the disease causes profound damage in many of their organ systems. Because they are asymptomatic, some patients do not adhere to their HCP's treatment recommendations. An effectively educated patient is more likely to modify their diet, exercise regularly, and take their medication properly in order to decrease their blood pressure. Educated patients are more likely to comply with instructions when they understand why they are important and are more likely to be satisfied patients. Therefore, it is the ultimate goal of all allied HCPs to both share information with their patients and to encourage them to make good decisions regarding their health.

Patient Education Involves More Than the Transfer of Information

A critical principle to consider with regard to patient education is that *knowledge* about health is necessary but not sufficient to influence health behaviors. If knowledge alone were indeed sufficient, there would likely be a decreased incidence of smoking (a cause of lung cancer and heart disease), excessive drinking (a cause of liver disease and neurologic disorders), obesity (a cause of type 2 diabetes, hypertension, and atherosclerosis), unplanned pregnancies, and sexually transmitted diseases. Furthermore, patients would be more likely to eat better and exercise more, which would serve to decrease hypercholesterolemia, heart disease, obesity, and osteoporosis.

Estimates of patient noncompliance with recommendations made by HCPs range from 50%–90%. As mentioned in the preceding chapter, some patients are at least somewhat knowledgeable about certain aspects of their health. However, with the increasing complexity of both health and disease, this is typically not the case. As a result, one cause of patient noncompliance with their HCP's recommendations is the lack of sufficient knowledge and understanding about their health problems and the recommended interventions. Another cause of noncompliance may be that many patients do not believe that it is possible for them to change a specific risk behavior. Therefore, it is essential that HCPs continually develop their ability to communicate with and educate their patients. In addition, the HCP must always be mindful that patients respond best when the HCP is encouraging, affirming, patient, and empathic toward them. A variety of strategies for effective patient education are presented in this chapter.

Approach to Patient Education

There are three steps in the approach to patient education:

- Assessment of the patient
- Design of the instruction
- Selection of teaching strategies and resources

Assessment of the Patient

To determine the type of instruction needed for a particular patient, four categories of variables must be assessed: contexts for the education, patient demographics, patient learning styles, and information and content to be included in the teaching session.

Situational context refers to the medical condition that creates the need for the instruction (e.g., chronic disease, surgery, acute illness). *Instructional context* refers to the environment in which the instruction will take place (e.g., doctor's office, hospital room, nursing home, outpatient clinic). There are a number of environmental factors of which the HCP should remain mindful, as they may influence the effectiveness of the instruction in a given environment. These include lighting, room temperature, the ability of the patient to hear the HCP clearly, distractions, and patient privacy.

Patient demographics refer to certain characteristics of the patient that may influence their response to the instruction. These characteristics include:

- Ethnicity and cultural background: A patient may prefer alternative therapies such as herbal medicine or acupuncture
- Socioeconomic background
- Patient's first language
- Age: Elderly patients may be more deferential toward HCPs
- Education level of the patient
- Healthcare background: Previous experiences with HCPs and healthcare institutions may influence a patient's perspective
- Physical and psychological conditions: Pain will certainly be distracting to a patient; anger, depression, or anxiety may also negatively

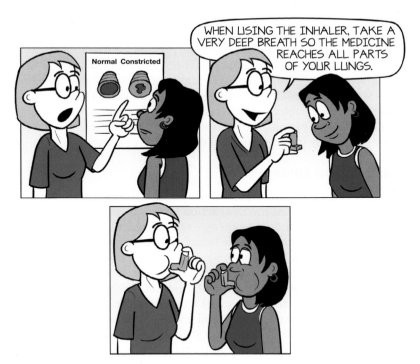

FIGURE 7-1. Three Types of Learners. All individuals have their own preferred learning styles. (**A**) Visual learners respond well to the use of pictures and anatomic models. (**B**) Auditory learners prefer to be engaged verbally in a discussion. (**C**) Kinesthetic learners learn by the physical demonstration of a task or technique.

influence the ability of the patient to focus on and absorb instruction provided for them

The greater the understanding that the HCP has regarding the patient and their perspective, the better the instruction can be adapted for the patient and the more effective the communication may be.

All individuals have their own preferred *learning styles*. In other words, they learn best in response to different teaching methods.

- *Visual learners* respond well to the use of pictures, diagrams, anatomic models, and literature.
- *Auditory learners* prefer to be engaged verbally with the use of questions and answers or discussion.
- *Kinesthetic learners* learn by the physical demonstration of a task or technique by the HCP followed by the practice of the technique by the patient.

The final component of the assessment phase is the *content analysis*. This is where the HCP determines what information should be included in the teaching session for the particular patient. Included in this is the identification of what information is essential as opposed to irrelevant or redundant, or simply interesting. In other words, the HCP must distinguish between *need-to-know* and *nice-to-know*. For example, the patient with asthma must be instructed on how to avoid precipitating factors, treatment options, and inhaler use. Anything else (e.g., prevalence of asthma in certain populations or the pathophysiologic mechanisms that trigger an attack) would be considered nonessential information. Other factors to consider regarding content selection include appropriateness of the material for a particular patient, the accuracy of the information, and the print size and readability of brochures and other forms of literature.

Design of the Instruction

During the design phase of patient education, the HCP organizes and structures the content of the instruction based upon the assessment of the patient. The HCP should begin by establishing behavioral objectives. These are specific and measurable behaviors that result from the instruction. For example, behavioral objectives for the obese patient would include establishing dietary practices and an exercise regimen that would result in weight loss at a rate of X pounds per week. A behavioral objective for the hypertensive patient would be taking medication properly 100% of the time to maintain blood pressure within the normal range.

The content should be organized so that the instruction is clear. The most important information should be provided in the beginning of the teaching session and repeated at the end. The HCP should provide support for the recommendation prior to listing any anticipated difficulties the patient may have in complying. For example, the beneficial effects of a particular medication should be described before the patient is warned of any potential side effects. Organization of the content is also determined by the type of instruction necessary. The use of an inhaler would involve procedural instruction, or a step-by-step method. The maintenance of blood glucose would involve instruction by topic or subject. In this case, the patient would be educated in the following topics: attention to diet, activity level, and insulin administration.

Selection of Teaching Strategies and Resources

The final step in the development of instruction is the selection of which strategies and resources to use with a particular patient. Teaching strategies will be determined by several factors including the type of information being taught, learner demographics, the patient's learning style, the learning environment, available resources and the HCP's comfort level with various teaching strategies. Resources may include the use of anatomic models or charts; written, visual or video materials; or any combination of these materials. Two types of media may be employed for patient teaching—that which is used during the teaching (e.g., models, videos) and that which may be used for patient reference at home (e.g., written materials).

TABLE 7-1

Summary of Strategies for Patient Instruction

- Welcome your patient warmly and introduce yourself.
- Appear knowledgeable, experienced, and confident.
- Ask the patient what they already know and think about the issue at hand.
- Be capable of communicating clearly and professionally using plain language.
- Observe nonverbal cues from the patient.
- Be aware of your own nonverbal behaviors toward the patient.
- Adapt the message according to the beliefs and concerns of the patient.
- Fully inform patients.
- Be specific.
- Recommend smaller changes in behavior instead of larger changes.
- Add new behaviors instead of eliminating old ones.
- Link new behaviors to the old ones.
- Use your "white coat."
- Encourage the patient to make a commitment.
- Repeat important information.
- Interact fully with the patient.
- Employ the technique of "demonstration and practice."
- Use a combination of instructional techniques.
- Ask the patient if they have any questions or concerns.
- Respect the patient's choices.

Strategies and Resources for Patient Instruction

Strategies and resources for designing and carrying out effective patient instruction include the following:

1 *Welcome your patient warmly and introduce yourself.* Establish a caring relationship by ensuring privacy and confidentiality, sitting at arm's length, and making appropriate eye contact (see Chapter 2).

2 *Appear knowledgeable, experienced, intelligent, and confident.* Remain patient and adaptable.

3 *Ask the patient what they already know and think about the issue at hand.* The American Academy on Physician and Patient suggests an "ask-tell-ask" framework. The HCP begins by asking the patient about their understanding and perspective of their condition as well as their expectations for outcomes with treatment. This will help the HCP to tailor explanations to the patient. The HCP then tells the patient about the diagnosis and management plan. Finally, the HCP invites the patient to ask any questions they may have.

4 *Be capable of communicating clearly and professionally using plain language.* Using plain language is not "dumbing down" or oversimplifying information to the point where it is inaccurate. Plain language is simply about clear and effective communication.

For example:

■ Keep sentences short and to the point.
■ Use the second person "you" instead of the third person "patients" or "people."

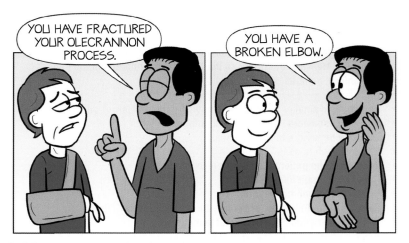

FIGURE 7-2. Clinical Terms versus Common Terms. Patients are unlikely to understand medical terminology. Whenever possible, substitute common terms for clinical terms to ensure patient understanding.

■ Limit the use of words consisting of three or more syllables. Use shorter words whenever possible.

■ Avoid excessive use of medical terminology as patients may be reluctant to say that they are confused or do not understand. If it is necessary to use it, explain the terms carefully to the patient and use them consistently. Be sure to confirm the patient's understanding of the terminology.

■ Whenever possible, substitute common terms for clinical terms. Examples of word substitutions include:

"Shot" instead of "intravenous or intramuscular injection"

"Pill" instead of "medication"

"Pain reliever" instead of "analgesic"

"Stomach upset" instead of "nausea"

"Heart attack" instead of "myocardial infarction"

"Stroke" instead of "cerebrovascular accident"

"Broken arm" instead of "fractured radius or ulna"

■ Use a professional speaking voice. This involves tone (e.g., calm, reassuring, authoritative), volume (e.g., appropriate for patient hearing), and pace (e.g., a rate at which the patient can hear and process the material). Use correct grammar.

 ROLE PLAY

Common Terms Versus Clinical Terms Used in Health Care

With a partner, make a list of at least five additional pairs of common terms and their associated clinical terms used in health care.

5 *Observe nonverbal cues from the patient.* This will help you to determine the patient's reaction to, and understanding of, the instruction.

6 *Be aware of your own nonverbal behaviors toward the patient* (See Chapter 2). Maintain a professional appearance, use appropriate eye contact, remain mindful of the use of hand gestures, and situate yourself at an appropriate distance from patient.

TABLE 7-2

Communicating Clearly Using Plain Language
• Keep sentences short and to the point.
• Use the second person "you."
• Limit the use of words with three or more syllables.
• Avoid excessive use of medical terminology.
• Substitute clinical terms with common terms.
• Use a professional speaking voice.

7 *Adapt the message according to the beliefs and concerns of the patient.* It is very important to identify a patient's perceptions of their health as well as their behaviors prior to providing instruction that is meant to change their behaviors. Examples of questions that may be directed toward patients to identify their beliefs and inform the design of the instruction include the following:

"What prevents you from quitting smoking?"
"What does hypertension mean to you?"
"What prevents you from using sunscreen?"
"What changes in your diet do you think that you could maintain?"
"Do you feel that you could incorporate some form of exercise into your routine?"

    The same message will not be effective for all patients; recommendations should take the patient's beliefs and concerns into account. For example, a patient may believe it to be impossible to quit smoking all at once. Instead, a less daunting recommendation could be to gradually cut down on the number of cigarettes consumed per day or to use a nicotine patch to reduce cravings.

8 *Fully inform patients.* In other words, the purposes and effects of interventions as well as when to expect these effects should be conveyed to the patient. For example, the therapeutic effects of antidepressants often take several weeks to become clinically apparent. A patient who expects this medication to act immediately like a pain reliever (e.g., aspirin, ibuprofen) may become discouraged and discontinue the treatment.

9 *Be specific.* Patients are likely to be more comfortable with instructions and, therefore, be more compliant when expectations are made very clear to them.

    Examples include the following: A patient scheduled for surgery in the morning should consume absolutely NO FOOD OR WATER after midnight. A patient who has been prescribed antibiotics must take ALL of the pills even after they are feeling better and have no symptoms.

10 *Recommend smaller changes in behavior instead of larger changes.* The patient who does not exercise at all may feel overwhelmed by a recommendation of 30 to 40 minutes of aerobic exercise four times per week. Instead, shorter bouts of exercise could be recommended initially. For example, the patient could begin with a ten minute walk three times per week. This exercise could be gradually increased by 5 minutes each week until the patient reaches the desired regimen.

11 *Add new behaviors instead of eliminating old ones.* A patient may not be able to avoid being outdoors and being exposed to the sun. Therefore, new recommended behaviors could include the proper use of sunscreen or wearing a hat and protective clothing.

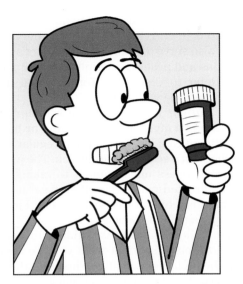

FIGURE 7-3. Link New Behaviors to Old Ones. Established behaviors, such as brushing one's teeth, will serve as reminders for new behaviors, such as taking medication.

12 *Link new behaviors to the old ones.* Begin by discussing the patient's daily routine. If a patient needs to take a medication two times per day, you could recommend that the medication be taken in the morning and evening when the patient brushes their teeth. Medication prescribed for three times per day could be taken with breakfast, lunch, and dinner. These established behaviors– brushing one's teeth and eating meals–will serve as reminders for the new behavior: taking medication.

13 *Use your "white coat."* Healthcare professionals are often regarded as authority figures, experts in their areas of specialty. Accordingly, patients have respect for their HCPs and consider their recommendations important. Therefore, the HCP should not be hesitant to make unpopular recommendations to their patients. It is possible to be firm with your patient while remaining encouraging and supportive. Examples include the following:

"You really must quit smoking. You will be able to breathe so much better."

"I want you to reduce the number of calories in your diet by 30%. Weight loss will make you feel better physically and emotionally."

"In order to better control your blood glucose, you need to avoid eating sweets randomly. Large swings in your blood glucose are contributing to your symptoms."

Emphasize the benefits of the recommendations. This will help to put any difficulties in carrying out the recommendations into perspective. It will also serve to enhance the patient's confidence in the recommendations and promote compliance. Use your "white coat" with caution. Refer to Chapter 3, for potential disadvantages in using the Directive Tone with patients.

14 *Encourage the patient to make a commitment.* For example, a patient who has had a myocardial infarction, or heart attack, must make a commitment to a low fat diet and regular exercise to minimize the likelihood of a second heart attack. The patient with hypertension or mental illness must commit to taking their prescribed medications as directed even when they have no symptoms. The diabetic patient must commit to checking their blood glucose regularly to better manage their diabetes.

15 *Repeat important information.* As with any form of instruction, it is often helpful to tell the patient what you are about to tell them, tell them, and then tell them what you just told them. Repetition of the material serves to reinforce the message.

16 *Fully interact with the patient.* Patient instruction will be more effective if the communication is two-way instead of one-way. Although the HCP is the expert in their area of specialty, the patient is the expert on their daily routine, their understanding of the nature of their illness and its treatment, and their anticipation of any problems in carrying out the recommendations made by the HCP. Therefore, the HCP should ask the patient any relevant questions that will help them to understand their patient's point of view. As the patient's perspective becomes clearer, the HCP may better adapt the message to the patient and the relationship between the HCP and the patient is strengthened. Furthermore, engaging the patient by asking them open-ended questions will increase their involvement and enable them to stay focused on the instruction at hand. For example, the HCP could ask the patient to repeat or summarize the instructions provided to them. In addition, the HCP will be able to verify that the patient has understood what they have been told. For example the HCP may say the following:

"Just to be sure that I was clear, can you tell me. . .?"
"In addition to developing a fever, when is it essential that you contact the doctor?"

17 *Employ the technique of "demonstration and practice."* Many individuals are kinesthetic learners and benefit from the demonstration of a medical device or instrument prior to practicing how to use it on their own. Instances where this would be beneficial include:
- Pediatric asthmatic patients and the use of inhalers
- Frail elderly patients and the use of walkers
- Diabetic patients and the use of glucometers

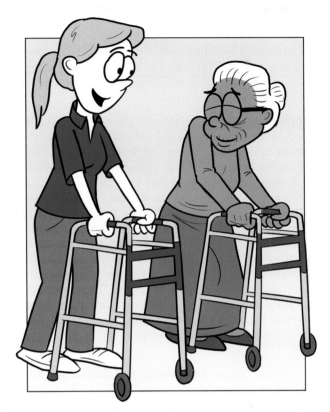

FIGURE 7-4. Demonstration and Practice. Kinesthetic learners benefit from the demonstration of a medical device or instrument prior to practicing how to use it on their own.

The HCP first demonstrates how to use the device or instrument while the patient observes. Then the patient practices how to use it while the HCP observes. In this way, the method of proper use is ensured and the patient will become more confident performing the task on their own.

18 *Use a combination of instructional techniques.* Patient instruction begins with effective verbal communication, which has been discussed extensively thus far in this chapter as well as previous chapters (Chapters 3 and 5). However, this verbal component of patient instruction may be significantly enhanced with the concurrent use of other teaching resources. Visual aids, such as anatomic models, charts, and drawings; audiovisual materials, such as videos; and written materials can clarify, support, and strengthen the message being conveyed by the HCP. For example, a model of the vertebral column may help the patient with a ruptured disk or a pinched nerve better understand the source of their pain and the nature of their treatment

plan. The patient with a blockage in a coronary artery may be treated by angioplasty. This patient's fear and anxiety may be reduced when they see the small actual size of the catheter (approximately 2 mm in diameter) used in the procedure. Remain mindful that any visual impairment on the part of the patient will limit the effectiveness of any visual aids.

Written materials regarding specific diseases or surgical procedures may be taken home by the patient for reference. However, it is important to note that the use of literature alone cannot take the place of direct interaction and communication between the HCP and the patient. According to the U.S. Department of Education, one in every five Americans cannot read the front page of a newspaper. Therefore, the patient's literacy level must be confirmed in order to avoid embarrassment on the part of the patient. If a patient simply smiles and nods when given medical literature, it may be a clue that they are not literate. Other clues to patient illiteracy may include making excuses when asked to read something (e.g., "I don't have my reading glasses with me.") and asking to return a filled-out form at a later time. A general guideline for the use of written materials with the overall patient population is not to exceed the fifth- to sixth-grade reading level.

ROLE PLAY	**Instructional Techniques and Resources**

With a partner—one patient and one HCP—provide patient instruction using more than one instructional technique or resource for each of the following scenarios.

- **A registered nurse instructs a 19-year-old college student who has conjunctivitis, or an eye infection, which will be treated with three drops placed in each eye.**
- **A medical assistant instructs a 24-year-old woman who has broken her tibia and is unsure of which bone this is.**

Discuss which technique or resource appeared more effective and why.

19 *Ask the patient if they have any questions or concerns.* The educational session may have raised additional questions or concerns on the part of the patient. In addition to asking the patient directly, look for nonverbal cues that the patient does not understand the instruction or that they may have concerns. Listen patiently and carefully and then respond clearly and empathically.

20 *Respect the patient's choices.* On occasion, the HCP may feel that the patient has not made the best choice in terms of treatment options or health behaviors. However, it is extremely important that the patient is always treated with respect and dignity.

Practices to Avoid During a Teaching Session

There are several practices or behaviors on the part of the HCP that may negatively impact the teaching session. These include the following:

- Repeatedly exiting and returning to the room or area where the instruction is taking place
- Encouraging interruptions from colleagues
- Avoiding eye contact by continuously writing notes while the patient is speaking
- Making negative facial expressions or using dismissive hand gestures toward the patient
- Making judgmental comments regarding the patient's concerns or choices

Patient instruction will be far more effective if the HCP is able to avoid or minimize the occurrence of these behaviors.

 Bad Practices

With a partner—one patient and one HCP—act out a teaching session regarding the use of pain medication following an appendectomy that includes several of the negative behaviors listed in the previous section. Discuss how these behaviors may affect the patient.

REVIEW QUESTIONS

OBJECTIVE QUESTIONS

1 Patients educated about their health are more likely to comply with recommendations made by their HCP. *(True or false?)*
2 The medical condition that creates the need for the instruction is referred to as the _____ context.
3 The most important information to be conveyed to the patient should be introduced at the end of the teaching session. *(True or false?)*
4 The beneficial effects of a recommendation should be described to the patient before they are warned of any potential difficulties or adverse effects. *(True or false?)*
5 Patient education is more effective when only clinical terms instead of common terms are used. *(True or false?)*
6 Patients are more likely to comply with recommendations for smaller changes in behavior rather than larger changes. *(True or false?)*

SHORT ANSWER QUESTIONS

1 Describe the three goals of patient education.
2 What are patient demographics? List the characteristics that may influence a patient's response to instruction.
3 Distinguish the three types of learning styles. Of these, which do you believe is your preferred learning style? Explain why.
4 What are behavioral objectives?
5 Why is two-way communication with a patient more effective than instruction that is one-way (from the HCP to the patient only)?

CLINICAL APPLICATIONS

1 Design a one-page brochure regarding a disease or disorder of your choice that will be used in your practice. Include the symptoms and the treatment options. Identify the qualities of your brochure that make it suitable for your particular patient.
2 A 5-year-old girl has come to your clinic with a terrible cold. Identify the behavioral objectives that you will teach her in order to avoid spreading her cold to the rest of her family.

Fundamental Writing Skills

The section in the writing skills chapter you should complete at the end of Chapter 7 is Section 10-7. You can find this section on pages 231–233.

SUGGESTED FURTHER READING

1. American Society of Health-System Pharmacists. ASHP guidelines on pharmacist-conducted patient education and counseling. *AJHP.*
2. Barrier PA, Li JT-C, Jensen NM. Two words to improve physician-patient communication: what else? *Mayo Clin Proc.* 2003;78:211–214.
3. Booth KA, Whicker LG, Wyman TD, et. al. *Medical Assisting, Administrative and Clinical Procedures Including Anatomy and Physiology.* 3rd ed. Boston: McGraw Hill; 2009.
4. Haynes RB. The teaching of patient education concepts on therapeutic compliance to medical students. *Bull NY Acad Med.* 1985;61(2):123–134.
5. Keller VF, Carroll JG. A new model for physician-patient communication. *Patient Educ Couns.* 1994;23:131–140.
6. Kelly-Heidenthal P. *Nursing Leadership & Management.* Clifton Park, NY: Thomson Delmar Learning; 2003.
7. Lorig K. Patient Education and Counseling for Prevention. Retrieved May 2010 from http://odphp.osophs.dhhs.gov/pubs/guidecps/text/iv_edu.txt.

8. McCann DP, Blossom HJ. The physician as a patient educator, from theory to practice. *West J Med.* 1990;153(1):44–49.

9. McGivney MS, Meyer SM, Duncan-Hewitt W, et. al. Medication therapy management: its relationship to patient counseling, disease management, and pharmaceutical care. *J Am Pharm Assoc.* 2007;47(5):620–628.

10. Stein T. Unhealthy mismatch, major gaps in Americans' understanding of medical concepts. *Nurse Week.* Retrieved May 2010 from http://www.nurseweek.com/features/00-05/literacy.html.

11. UC Davis Center for Nursing Education. *Guidelines for preparing patient education handouts.* Retrieved May 2010 from http://www.ucdmc.ucdavis.edu/cne/health_education/guide.html.

12. U.S. Department of Health and Human Services, Office of Disease Prevention and Health Promotion, Plain language: A promising strategy for clearly communicating health information and improving health literacy. Retrieved May 2010 from http://www.health.gov/communication/literacy/plainlanguage/PlainLanguage.htm.

13. World Health Organization. *Integrating STI/RTI Care for Reproductive Health, Sexually Transmitted and Other Reproductive Tract Infections, A Guide to Essential Practice.* Retrieved May 2010 from http://who.int/reproductive-health/publications/rtis_gep/rtis_gep.pdf.

8

CULTURAL SENSITIVITY IN HEALTHCARE COMMUNICATION

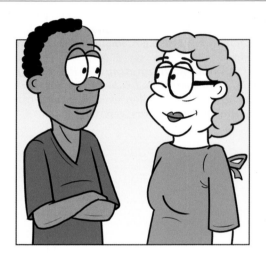

OBJECTIVES

- Discuss the ways in which our society is becoming more multicultural and ethnically diverse
- Explain the documented disparity that ethnic and racial minorities perceive in the quality and availability of health care
- Define cultural competence and explain the need for it on the part of HCPs
- Describe two models on developing cultural competence
- Discuss nonverbal communication between cultures
- Explain the responsibilities of all healthcare providers under the National Standards for Culturally and Linguistically Appropriate Services in Health Care (CLAS)
- Discuss the need for and the use of interpreters

When you get down to it, any communication between a healthcare professional (HCP) and a patient is a form of cross-cultural communication. On the one side, the HCP approaches the encounter from the culture of the healthcare provider, or the one who treats someone for healthcare reasons. On the other, the patient comes to the encounter from the very different culture of healthcare recipient, or the one who is treated for healthcare reasons. Each wants to get to the same destination—a positive patient outcome—but each comes from a different starting place: The HCP comes from an understanding of what causes the illness from which the patient suffers, and the patient comes from an experience of the symptoms of the illness. The main purpose of all of the other chapters in this book is to help you as an HCP bridge this cultural divide and communicate effectively with patients. The main purpose of this particular chapter on cultural sensitivity in health care is to help you understand how HCP–patient communication can best work in the context of the broader cultural differences of ethnicity, race, and language.

A More Multicultural and Ethnically Diverse Society

Immigration and birth patterns are rapidly changing the cultural and ethnic make-up of the United States and other Western countries. According to the U.S. Census Bureau, in 2008 the population of the United States

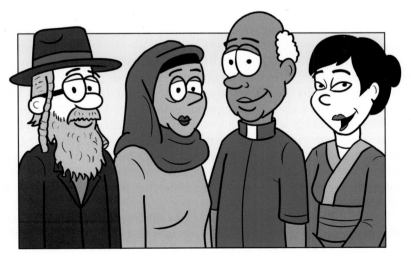

FIGURE 8-1. A More Multicultural and Ethnically Diverse Society. Immigration and birth patterns are rapidly changing the cultural and ethnic makeup of the United States and other Western countries.

was 66% non-Hispanic white, just over 14% Hispanic, almost 13% black, and just over 4% Asian. By 2050, the Hispanic and Asian populations should nearly triple, whereas the black population should grow by 60%. The non-Hispanic white population will become a much smaller segment of the U.S. population, comprising only 46% of the total. Among all of these groups there exist what sociologists call co-cultures, that is, smaller groups within every group broken down by age, ethnicity, gender, sexual orientation, religion, occupation, physical disability, or even leisure activity. Clearly, an HCP in the 21st century needs to develop an understanding of the complex diversity that will characterize society as well as a strong cultural sensitivity—or cultural competence, as it is often called—to work effectively with such a population. Indeed, it has become clear that cultural competence is an important—perhaps *the* most important—competency an effective communicator can possess.

Disparities in Treatment and Access to Health Care

There is significant, documented evidence to indicate that racial and ethnic minorities receive lower quality, and poorer access to, health care. These disparities, or differences, exist independently of such socioeconomic factors as income level, access to medical insurance, and geographical proximity to healthcare facilities. Studies have shown that cardiovascular disease, cancer, and HIV are just three of the diseases for which minority patients are likely to experience disparities in healthcare access and treatment, frequently resulting in poorer patient outcomes.

Members of these minority groups also perceive these differences. For example, more than half of African American respondents on a 2006 Kaiser Family Foundation survey said that they believed that racial differences existed in access to health care. A full 55% believed that they were likely to receive lower quality health care than whites. On the same survey, nearly half of all Latinos, or 48%, said that they also believed they would receive lower quality health care than white patients. Such perceptions, based in part on reality, lead to despair among these patient groups of ever receiving an adequate range of treatment options.

Today, professionals throughout the healthcare industry—from hospital and insurance executives to physicians and nurses to higher education administrators to their allied health graduates (one of whom you will soon be)—are coming to recognize that cultural competence is absolutely necessary to effective communication with patients and other members of the healthcare team.

Defining Cultural Competence and Some Ideas about It

The American Medical Association (AMA) has defined cultural competence as "the knowledge and interpersonal skills that allow providers to understand, appreciate, and work with individuals from cultures other than their own. It involves an awareness and acceptance of cultural differences; self-awareness; knowledge of the patient's culture; and adaptation of skills." We should note that this is one of many definitions of cultural competence; there is no universally agreed-upon definition of the term. However, most of the definitions in use today contain the idea that cultural competence requires an understanding of one's own culture and background in order to understand other cultures. Moreover, there is no agreed-upon best method or path for an HCP to learn cultural competence. A brief look at two models for acquiring these interpersonal skills and knowledge will help us understand more about the process.

I. The Volcano Model—"The Process of Cultural Competence in the Delivery of Healthcare Services"

This model, developed by Josepha Campinha-Bacote, defines cultural competence as "the process in which the HCP continually strives to achieve the ability and availability to effectively work within the cultural context of the client (family, individual, or community). It is a process of *becoming* culturally competent, not *being* culturally competent" (Campinha-Bacote). This process contains the following five steps:

1 Cultural Awareness. This is the process of looking closely and honestly at your own biases toward other cultures, as well as examining your own cultural background. Cultural awareness includes an awareness that racism and other forms of discrimination exist in healthcare delivery;

2 Cultural Knowledge. This is the process of seeking a thorough understanding of the attitudes and beliefs of other cultural and ethnic groups, as well as the health conditions and diseases that exist among diverse ethnic groups;

3 Cultural Skill. This is the ability to accurately understand the cultural details surrounding the patient's presenting problem and to physically assess the patient within the context of their culture;

4 Cultural Encounter. This is when the HCP actively seeks face-to-face encounters with members of other cultures in order to better understand the HCP's own beliefs about other cultures and to prevent stereotyping;

5 Cultural Desire. This is the all-important desire of the HCP to become more culturally knowledgeable and skillful. It is important

Box 8-1 Examples (and Frequent Generalizations) of Some Communication Gestures and Their Meanings Among Non-Hispanic Whites and African Americans

Activity/Gesture	Non-Hispanic White	African American
Touching another person's hair	Touching another person's hair is a sign of affection.	Touching another person's hair is generally considered offensive.
Asking personal questions	Inquiring about jobs, family, and other personal matters at a first meeting is considered friendly.	Asking personal questions of a person at a first meeting may be considered improper, even intrusive.
Using direct questions	Use of direct questions for personal information is generally considered normal.	Use of direct questions can be considered harassment.
Interrupting conversations	Normative rules on taking turns in conversation dictate that one person has the floor until they have finished.	"Breaking in" during conversation by participants is normally tolerated. Competition for the floor is granted by the group to the person who is most assertive.
Listening in and jumping into the conversations of others	Adding points of information or insights to a conversation in which one is not engaged can be considered helpful.	Conversations are regarded as private between the recognized participants; "butting in" may be considered eavesdropping and is usually not tolerated.
The use of the expression "You people"	The use of the expression "you people" is tolerated.	The use of the expression "you people" is typically considered pejorative and even racist.
Eye contact when listening	Listeners are expected to look at a speaker directly to indicate respect and attention.	Listeners are expected to avert eyes to indicate respect and attention.
Eye contact when speaking	Speakers are expected to flit and even avert eyes, especially in informal speaking situations.	Speakers are expected to look at listeners directly in the eye.
Including a minority person in an activity	Including a minority person in group activities is considered democratic.	Purposely including a minority person in group activities is considered tokenism.
Speaking like another group	Borrowing language forms from another group is permissible and even encouraged.	An outsider talking "Black" is considered to be making an insult.
Showing emotions	Showing emotions during conflict is perceived as the beginning of a "fight" and obstacle to conflict resolution.	Showing emotions during conflict is perceived as honesty and the first step toward the resolution of a problem.

(Source: *Cross Cultural Communication—an Essential Dimension of Effective Education*)

to emphasize that this has to be something the HCP genuinely wants to do instead of merely a need to fulfill a job requirement.

II. The Cultural Competence Continuum

This model, created by researchers at Georgetown University's Child Development Center, describes a range of six points on a continuum, or scale, of cultural competence. See Figure 8-2. These include the following:

1 Cultural Destructiveness. This point on the scale is characterized by attitudes, policies, structures, and practices by an individual or within a system or organization that are destructive to members of a cultural group. This can refer to openly hostile racist behavior on the part of a single person or to a destructive act committed by a group or institution against a different cultural group. A notorious example of such cultural destructiveness was the Tuskegee Experiments begun in the 1930s, in which American government researchers recruited African American men who had been infected with syphilis and then left them untreated in order to observe them and the progression of their disease. Other examples exist, too. As recently as October 2010, the United States government revealed that in the 1940s researchers from the U.S. Public Health Service deliberately and secretly infected with syphilis up to 700 men living in Guatemala in order test the effectiveness of penicillin–which was a relatively new drug at the time–in treating the disease. U.S. Secretary of State Hillary Clinton and Secretary of Health and Human Services Kathleen

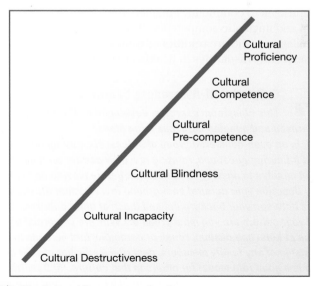

FIGURE 8-2. **The Cultural Competence Continuum.**

Sebelius publicly apologized to the government of Guatemala for what they called the "clearly unethical" experiments.

2 Cultural Incapacity. This point describes the inability of an individual or institution to respond effectively to the needs and interests of culturally and linguistically diverse groups. For example, a pharmacy manager in a predominantly white neighborhood who is so afraid of displeasing customers that he becomes reluctant to hire qualified candidates for an open pharmacist job because of skin color or strong accent is demonstrating real cultural incapacity.

3 Cultural Blindness. This describes the stance taken by many people or institutions of viewing and treating all people from different cultures as if they were the same. An HCP who does not recognize that women from some groups, such as Muslims or Latinas, may feel deeply uncomfortable being touched by a stranger, particularly a male stranger, suffers from cultural blindness.

4 Cultural Precompetence. This point on the continuum describes a level of awareness by people or institutions of their capacity for growth in responding effectively to culturally and linguistically diverse groups. This is true for many hospitals and healthcare organizations that recognize the need to provide cultural training to their employees.

5 Cultural Competence. This term describes individuals or institutions that demonstrate an acceptance and respect for cultural differences.

6 Cultural Proficiency. This describes individuals or institutions that have a high regard for diverse culture and use this ethical stance as a foundation to guide their endeavors. From a desire to do so, such individuals actively pursue the development of their own cultural competence and seek to continually enhance their organization's capacities in cultural and linguistic competence. They advocate with, and on behalf of, populations who are traditionally underserved, and they also work to eliminate any disparities in healthcare availability and treatment.

> **ROLE PLAY**   **Cultural Self-Awareness Exercise**
>
> *This classroom exercise, developed by Gary Coombs and Yolanda Sarason and adapted here, has three steps.*
>
> *Step I: In an even-numbered group of at least six, pair up and answer each of the following questions, rotating to a new partner with each question. Allow 3 to 4 minutes to answer each question before moving on to the next partner. (1) Describe your cultural background in a way that illustrates the differences between your background and those of other cultures. (2) What aspects of your culture are you most proud of? Why are you proud of these? (3) Describe at least one custom, ritual, or ceremony that belongs to your culture. (4) Outside of any family members, describe a member of your cultural group who is a good role model for others in that culture. (5) Describe a situation in which you felt out of place as a result of being different from others.*

Step II: Now, choose a culture other than your own, and pretend that you are a member of that other culture. Rotating through the group as you did in Step I, answer the same five questions from the standpoint of someone from that other culture.

Step III: Gather together again as a class and discuss the following questions. Was it easy or hard to answer the questions from the standpoint of a culture different from yours? Why? Would it have been easier if you had chosen yet another culture? Did you feel uncomfortable trying to imagine answering the questions for another culture? Why? Do your believe members of that other culture would find your answers accurate?

Nonverbal Communication in Cross-Cultural Contexts

Nonverbal communication is the primary means of expression for all cultures, and the meanings of different forms of nonverbal communication can vary greatly among different cultures. Even within a given culture, nonverbal communication can vary from individual to individual, depending upon age, education, gender, socioeconomic status, or geographic background. As an HCP who will work in an increasingly diverse workplace, you should be aware that many forms of nonverbal communication that seem absolutely clear to you may in fact mean very different

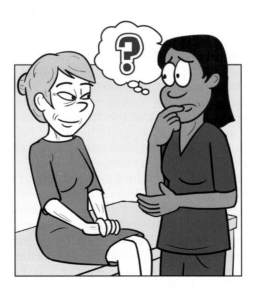

FIGURE 8-3. Nonverbal Communication between Different Cultures. A smile is a powerful form of nonverbal communication and can mean different things to members of different cultures. Sometimes a smile may be difficult to interpret.

things to people from other cultures, increasing the chances for misunderstanding. It is important for HCPs to be aware of differences and to be cautious in both interpreting and conveying nonverbal communication. Some examples of areas in which such misunderstanding may occur include the following:

- Facial Expression. Facial expressions play an important part of any interpersonal communication, but interpreting the exact meaning of facial expressions can be difficult when you are communicating across cultures. As noted previously in Chapter 2, there exist six facial expressions that are considered universal: happiness, sadness, fear, anger, disgust, and surprise. However, although any of these facial expressions may result from an emotion felt by an individual, different cultures have different norms that dictate when, where, how, and to whom some facial expressions are appropriate to display. Here follow just a couple examples to illustrate the point:
  - The Smile—Everyone knows how to smile. However, not all the members of all cultures smile for the same reason, and not all cultures believe that smiling is appropriate in the same situations. Smiling is an expression of happiness in American culture. Germans also smile as an indication of happiness, but only smile when with people they know closely and really like. In many Asian cultures the smile can mean something else altogether. Some Chinese, for example, may smile when they are discussing something sad or uncomfortable. In Japanese culture, a smile can be used to hide an emotion or to avoid answering a question. Even within Japanese culture there can be differences. For instance, a person of lower social status in Japan may use a smile when taking orders from a superior when in fact they feel anger or contempt toward the superior. In Korean culture, smiling too much can be interpreted as the sign of a shallow person, leading many Koreans to smile less in public. One scholar notes that this "lack of smiling by Koreans has often been interpreted as a sign of hostility." People in Thailand, however, smile a lot, leading that country to be called "The Land of Smiles" by some students of culture.
  - Crying or Expressions of Grief and Sadness—Crying and other expressions of grief and sadness are also specific to various cultures. White American men, for example, often suppress these expressions in public. Men of Chinese, Japanese, and Korean cultures also resist displaying these emotions through facial expressions, whereas men from Mediterranean cultures, such as Greek and Italian, readily display these emotions and even exaggerate them. The HCP with effective communication skills will recognize that some cultures may value a stoic affect, whereas others may encourage a more emotional expression.

Box 8-2 Forms of Nonverbal Communication Among Asians

Gesture/ Activity	Japanese	Chinese	Korean	Indian
Greeting	Graceful bow, will shake hands among Westerners.	Shaking hands is the custom.	Graceful bow, will shake hands among Westerners.	The traditional *Namaste*—a greeting in which the palms are pressed together chest-high, accompanied by a slight bow.
Eye Contact	Individuals can feel uncomfortable with sustained, direct eye contact.	People can feel that prolonged, direct eye contact is a sign of disrespect. In crowded situations, Chinese people will avoid eye contact to maintain privacy.	Direct eye contact is common among friends, but disrespectful for a young South Korean to make prolonged direct eye contact with an older person or authority figure.	Sustained, direct eye contact can be interpreted as a sign of disrespect, especially when directed at an older person.
Personal Space	When possible, individuals provide each other with plenty of personal space; however, in tight public spaces (e.g., train stations) personal space is understood to be much smaller.	People stand close together when talking with each other.	Individuals stand close together when talking with each other.	People stand close together when talking with each other.

(Sources: *Gestures: Do's and Taboos of Body Language around the World* and *Multicultural Manners*)

■ Eye Contact—Eye contact is an important form of nonverbal communication, and like facial expression, it can mean different things in different cultures. In white American culture, direct eye contact is expected of someone who is listening to a speaker, whereas a speaker is expected to make frequent but flitting eye contact. Moreover, in white American culture, a speaker who makes constant direct eye contact with the listener can be interpreted as hostile or angry. Among African Americans, a listener will frequently avert their eyes when listening to indicate respect and attention, whereas a speaker in African American culture will look a listener directly in the eye. In some cultures, making direct eye contact is a sign of disrespect. Members of both Chinese and Japanese cultures, for instance, avoid extended direct eye contact with strangers and authority figures out of respect and deference. American Indians often stare at the floor during a conversation to indicate that they are listening closely to the speaker. In other cultures, such as those from Latin America, the Arab world, or southern Europe, direct eye contact is appropriate and expected of a person in authority, such as an HCP.

■ Touching—As an HCP, you will frequently need to touch patients simply to do your job. However, you must remain aware that touching another person can have very different meanings to members of different cultures. The members of some cultures, such as white American culture, are accustomed to being touched by their HCPs during the process of a visit to the doctor's office, while members of other cultures may feel deeply uncomfortable at the prospect of being touched by the HCP. Members of Latino cultures, for instance, engage in frequent touching when socializing but can feel uneasy when being touched by a medical professional. Latino women may resist exposing their bodies to male or female HCPs, and can become very embarrassed during pelvic examinations. People from Asian cultures may also feel uncomfortable about being touched, especially on the head. To touch another person's head can be considered offensive by some people from these cultures, as such a gesture can even have a religious meaning. One observer notes that "many Asian people believe the head houses the soul. Therefore, when another person touches their head, it places them in jeopardy." Although Arab men may engage in frequent touching and even handholding with other Arab men as a sign of friendship with no sexual connotation at all, Muslim women can feel so uncomfortable as to refuse touch by any male outside of marriage, including their HCPs.

■ Handshaking—This form of touch and its meaning can also vary greatly from culture to culture. American culture commonly uses the handshake as a form of greeting with friends and strangers. But other cultures have complex views of handshaking. Many Chinese, for instance, will use a handshake to greet a Westerner, but any other contact may be considered inappropriate. In Arab culture, men will shake using their right hands–to use the left hand to greet someone is a harsh social insult, as members of this culture use only the left hand to engage in basic biological and hygienic functions.

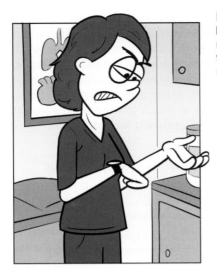

FIGURE 8-4. Nonverbal Communication between Different Cultures. Attitudes and responses to such nonverbal communication as punctuality are different in different cultures.

■ Time—How we use time communicates a lot about us. For example, if you are 45 minutes late for an appointment and do not offer any apology or explanation, you are sending a clear message about yourself. If you arrive 45 minutes late and are so preoccupied with apologies as to neglect the reason for your appointment, you are sending a very different message about yourself. As an HCP, you will come into contact with patients from varying cultures who will have strikingly different ideas about time and its use. Of special significance to your interaction as an HCP with members of other cultures are the ways differing attitudes can impact views of punctuality and the pace at which time is lived.

　■ Punctuality—American culture views punctuality as a virtue, a characteristic of a person who behaves appropriately when interacting with others. Many Americans would be surprised to learn, however, that other cultures consider punctuality to be not a virtue but a fault, and in some cases inconsiderate or even rude. In much of Latin America, arriving late for an appointment is considered a sign of respect. In Chile, showing up on time for a social event is an act of rudeness. In Spain, one observer has noted, people believe that "punctuality messes up schedules." Germans, however, would consider such lateness intolerable. A practicing HCP should be aware of the many different accepted ideas of punctuality when interacting with people of other cultures.

　■ The Pace of Time—To most of the world, Americans always seem to be in a hurry. They cannot wait to finish what they are doing now so that they can move on to the next task. American children hear from an early age that they shouldn't "dawdle" or waste time, and that "there's no time like the present." Other cultures from around the world, however, do not understand what the rush is. When interacting with a patient, an American HCP may believe that small talk has its place in building rapport with patients but that is all. Members from other cultures, from Latinos to Asians to Arabs, would expect their HCP to spend significant time getting to know them through small talk. Such groups may also expect the HCP to explain any disease and treatment at much greater length and in more detail than their American counterparts would.

Box 8-3 Forms of Nonverbal Communication Among Latin Americans

Gesture/ Activity	Mexicans	Brazilians	Puerto Ricans	Venezuelans
Greeting	A warm, some-what soft handshake among both men and women. After a second or third meeting, men may greet with the *abrazo*, or embrace, along with a few pats on the back.	A strong, warm handshake is the traditional greeting. Among friends, men may engage in the *abraço*, or embrace.	The handshake is the custom-ary greeting. Old friends may engage in *abrazo*.	A warm, gentle handshake. Men who know each other well may use the *abrazo*. Men and women friends who are close may kiss, and women friends will hug and kiss on the cheeks.
Eye Contact	Prolonged, direct eye contact can suggest disrespect.	Sustained, direct eye contact is important.	Prolonged eye contact can suggest disrespect.	Good eye con-tact during social and business conversations is considered important and polite.
Personal Space	Individuals stand close together when speaking to one another.	Individuals stand close together when speaking to one another.	People stand close together in social settings. To move back or away during a conversation may be consid-ered offensive.	Individuals stand close together when socializing.

(Sources: *Gestures: Do's and Taboos of Body Language around the World* and *Multicultural Manners*)

The National Standards on Culturally and Linguistically Appropriate Services (CLAS)

Written and published by the Office of Minority Health (OMH) in the U.S. Department of Health and Human Services, these standards are intended primarily for healthcare organizations, but they can also help individual healthcare providers make their practices more culturally and linguistically accessible to patients from all cultures. Although not legally binding—that is, they are not required by law—these standards should be practiced at all levels of patient care to ensure that the different cultural communities served have sufficient access to appropriate care.

TABLE 8-1

U.S. Department of Health and Human Services—Office of Minority Health National Standards on Culturally and Linguistically Appropriate Services (CLAS)

Standard 1
Healthcare organizations should ensure that patients/consumers receive from all staff members effective, understandable, and respectful care that is provided in a manner compatible with their cultural health beliefs and practices and preferred language.

Standard 2
Healthcare organizations should implement strategies to recruit, retain, and promote at all levels of the organization a diverse staff and leadership that are representative of the demographic characteristics of the service area.

Standard 3
Healthcare organizations should ensure that staff at all levels and across all disciplines receive ongoing education and training in culturally and linguistically appropriate service delivery.

Standard 4
Healthcare organizations must offer and provide language assistance services, including bilingual staff and interpreter services, at no cost to each patient/consumer with limited English proficiency at all points of contact, in a timely manner during all hours of operation.

Standard 5
Healthcare organizations must provide to patients/consumers in their preferred language both verbal offers and written notices informing them of their right to receive language assistance services.

Standard 6
Healthcare organizations must assure the competence of language assistance provided to limited English proficient patients/consumers by interpreters and bilingual staff. Family and friends should not be used to provide interpretation services (except on request by the patient/consumer).

(continued)

TABLE 8-1 *(Continued)*

U.S. Department of Health and Human Services—Office of Minority Health National Standards on Culturally and Linguistically Appropriate Services (CLAS)

Standard 7
Healthcare organizations must make available easily understood patient-related materials and post signage in the languages of the commonly encountered groups and/or groups represented in the service area.

Standard 8
Healthcare organizations should develop, implement, and promote a written strategic plan that outlines clear goals, policies, operational plans, and management accountability/oversight mechanisms to provide culturally and linguistically appropriate services.

Standard 9
Healthcare organizations should conduct initial and ongoing organizational self-assessments of CLAS-related activities and are encouraged to integrate cultural and linguistic competence-related measures into their internal audits, performance improvement programs, patient satisfaction assessments, and outcomes-based evaluations.

Standard 10
Healthcare organizations should ensure that data on the individual patient's/consumer's race, ethnicity, and spoken and written language are collected in health records, integrated into the organization's management information systems, and periodically updated.

Standard 11
Healthcare organizations should maintain a current demographic, cultural, and epidemiological profile of the community as well as a needs assessment to accurately plan for and implement services that respond to the cultural and linguistic characteristics of the service area.

Standard 12
Healthcare organizations should develop participatory, collaborative partnerships with communities and utilize a variety of formal and informal mechanisms to facilitate community and patient/consumer involvement in designing and implementing CLAS-related activities.

Standard 13
Healthcare organizations should ensure that conflict and grievance resolution processes are culturally and linguistically sensitive and capable of identifying, preventing, and resolving cross-cultural conflicts or complaints by patients/consumers.

Standard 14
Healthcare organizations are encouraged to regularly make available to the public information about their progress and successful innovations in implementing the CLAS standards and to provide public notice in their communities about the availability of this information.

The 14 standards are organized by themes: Culturally Competent Care (Standards 1–3), Language Access Services (Standards 4–7), and Organizational Supports for Cultural Competence (Standards 8–14).

Within this framework, standards are categorized by varying levels of stringency: mandates, guidelines, and recommendations as follows:

- Some of these standards—called CLAS *mandates*—are current Federal requirements for all recipients of Federal funds (Standards 4–7).
- Others—called CLAS *guidelines*—are activities recommended by the Department of Health and Human Services for adoption as mandates by Federal, State, and national accrediting agencies (Standards 1–3, and 8–13).
- CLAS *recommendations* are suggested by OMH for voluntary adoption by healthcare organizations (Standard 14).

Tips for Improving Cross-Cultural Communication between the HCP and Patient

These tips for helping you communicate with members of cultures different from your own are based primarily on common sense and practicality. They are intended to help you serve your patients' healthcare needs while treating those patients with respect and dignity.

1. *Do not treat the patient in the same manner you would want to be treated.* "Do unto others as you would have them do unto you" does not necessarily hold in cross-cultural communication. Different cultures have different rules for appropriate, polite behavior. Try to understand and be sensitive to each patient's cultural values while

TABLE 8-2

Tips for Improving Cross-Cultural Communication Between HCP and Patient

- Do not treat the patient in the same manner you would want to be treated.
- Begin by being more formal with patients who were born in another culture.
- Do not worry if the patient fails to look you directly in the eye or ask questions about the treatment.
- Do not assume anything about the patient's ideas about how to maintain good health, what causes illness, or ways to prevent or cure illness. When a patient is ill, be sure to ask what they believe caused the illness.
- Ask the patient how they prefer to make their medical decisions.
- Never assume that the patient is familiar with any particular type of medical test or procedure.

Paraphrasing Effectively for a Patient Who is Limited-English-Speaking

With two other classmates, where one is the HCP, one the patient, and one an observer, act out the following scenario while using Tips 4, 5, and 6. An HCP listens to a patient's description of recurring knee pain when the patient takes part in some sport or physical activity (let the patient decide what activity). The HCP should then paraphrase what the patient has said in concise, clear, idiom-free English. What were some of the problems that the observer noticed? How could this be done more effectively?

7 *Check to see that the patient understands the concepts behind the words*—Limited-English-speaking patients may interpret even the simplest instructions in ways you do not intend or foresee. A simple instruction such as "wash the wound regularly" may elicit completely different responses from members of different cultures who have different conceptions of what "regularly" means. To some, the word "regularly" may mean the frequency of washing, whereas to others it may indicate the manner of washing.

 Clearly Explaining What the HCP Means by a Word Like "Regularly"

With a partner, identify examples of other words that can be ambiguous to patients and find more suitable substitutes.

TABLE 8-4

Summary of Strategies for Using a Medical Interpreter

- Brief the interpreter.
- Look at the patient and address them directly.
- Explain information and ask questions in more than one way.
- Avoid long, complicated sentences.
- Break up what you have to say into short segments.
- Allow the interpreter time to think.
- Do not interrupt the interpreter.
- Remember that English is a direct language.
- Use appropriate facial expressions and gestures and take advantage of the interpreter's speaking time to examine those of the patient.
- Remember that the culture of the second language may cause the interpreter to modify what you or the patient has said.

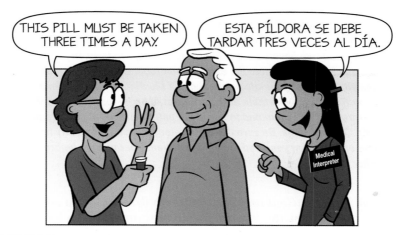

FIGURE 8-5. The Need for a Medical Interpreter. The services of an interpreter may be necessary for providing care to some patients whose understanding of English is minimal. Knowing how to utilize a medical interpreter effectively can take some practice.

8 *Avoid questions that can elicit a simple yes or no*—A "yes" or "no" answer to such questions tells you only that the patient has heard the question. Verify that the patient understands by asking questions that ask *what, when, where,* and *how.* For example, when a patient with limited-English-speaking skills comes into your department complaining of pain, be sure to ask *what* the patient was doing and *when* they first experienced the pain. Ask the patient to describe exactly *where* the pain is. Follow up with *how* the pain feels, that is, is the pain sharp, dull, localized?

The Need for a Medical Interpreter

You will need the services of an interpreter for providing care to some patients whose understanding of English is minimal. Knowing how to utilize a medical interpreter effectively can take some practice, as the process can feel confusing to first-timers who may not even be sure who to speak to. Below is a list of suggestions to follow when working with an interpreter:

1 *Brief the interpreter*—Before working with the patient, summarize for the interpreter the key information you want to convey. Have a preconference with the interpreter, providing them with a list of the topics and questions you intend to discuss with the patient.

Briefing the Interpreter

With three other classmates, where one is the HCP, one the interpreter, and two observers, act out the following scenario. In just a few minutes, the HCP must go into the examination room with the interpreter to take the vital signs of a female patient who is Muslim. You can assume the patient will feel uncomfortable at the prospect of being touched. Explain to the interpreter what you intend to say to the patient and what you intend to do in taking the vital signs. Be sure the interpreter understands clearly how you will proceed and that you need to gain the patient's permission before you touch her.

2 *Look at the patient and address them directly*—You are serving the patient, not the interpreter. It is appropriate to look at the patient.

ROLE PLAY **Addressing a Patient When an Interpreter is Present**

With three classmates, where one is the HCP, one the patient, one the interpreter, and one an observer, act out the scenario of actually taking the patient's vital signs as described in the preceding role play. The HCP should be sure to look at the patient when you address her and not at the interpreter. (Remember that for this role play you will all probably be speaking English.) Discuss what worked? What practices would be inappropriate and impair communication?

3 *Explain information and ask questions in more than one way*— You should never be afraid of repeating yourself. Rephrasing what you may have already said in a new way may help avoid any misunderstanding by the patient.

ROLE PLAY **Giving Instructions and Helping the Patient Using Different Words**

With a partner, where one is a nurse practitioner and the other a patient, act out the following scenario. The pharmacy technician must explain to the patient how they should apply a cortisone ointment to the scalp near the hairline. Practice explaining these instructions in more than one way, each time using different words. What practices worked? Were there any that impaired communication?

4 *Avoid long, complicated sentences*—To minimize the possibility of inaccurate interpretation, always be concise and direct when speaking to the patient.

5 *Break up what you have to say into short segments*—Avoid talking for more than a few sentences without letting the interpreter explain what you have said to the patient.

6 *Allow the interpreter time to think*—A professionally trained interpreter will try to capture the gist, or essence, of what you mean rather than simply translating word for word what you say. This may take time.

Working with the Medical Interpreter to Explain to the Patient How to Perform a Procedure

With two to three classmates, where one is the HCP, one the patient, one the interpreter and one an observer, act out the following scenario. The HCP must explain to the patient through the interpreter the need for, and manner of, performing a procedure (for example, collecting a urine sample or flossing one's teeth). Using the advice from Tips 3–6, explain in detail to the patient what is necessary. Remember to speak clearly and in short segments, and remember to give the interpreter time to think. (Keep in mind that all three of you will probably be speaking English.) Discuss what was effective in facilitating communication with the patient. What impaired communication?

7 *Do not interrupt the interpreter*—Doing this can confuse the interpreter's communication to the patient and also undermine their authority in the eyes of the patient.

8 *Remember that English is a direct language*—The interpreter can take longer to say in the second language what you have said in English because the second language may use constructions or expressions that are longer. Moreover, the patient may take longer to speak back to the interpreter in response.

9 *Use appropriate facial expressions and gestures and take advantage of the interpreter's speaking time to examine those of the patient*—Seat yourself or stand in such a way so that you, the patient, and the interpreter can all see each other. When you speak, use appropriate facial expressions and gestures so that the interpreter and patient can use these for understanding. Take advantage of the time during which the interpreter and patient speak to observe the patient's facial expressions and gestures. These can help you in understanding their meaning.

10 *Remember that the culture of the second language may cause the interpreter to modify what you or the patient has said*—Different cultures may approach a discussion of delicate issues such as sex or death differently and may, therefore, have widely varying expressions and manners for communicating on such topics.

REVIEW QUESTIONS

OBJECTIVE QUESTIONS

1 The expression "cultural competence" describes the ability to name the different cultures on the different continents of the world. *(True or False?)*

2 African Americans in general agree that there are no differences between the quality and availability of health care that they receive and what non-Hispanic whites receive. *(True or False?)*

3 The non-Hispanic white population in the United States is the fastest growing segment of the population. *(True or False?)*

4 A patient who is listening to the HCP but looking at the floor may not be showing disrespect and disagreement. *(True or False?)*

5 It is important to know something of your own cultural background and biases when learning to be more competent in working with other cultures. *(True or False?)*

6 A smile on the face of any person must always mean that they are happy. *(True or False?)*

7 A pharmacy manager who hires people of different cultures and then wants them to learn to act and sound just like him is not demonstrating cultural competence. *(True or False?)*

8 You should look at and address the patient when using a medical interpreter. *(True or False?)*

9 It is a good idea to quickly interrupt a medical interpreter if you believe they have slightly changed the phrasing of instructions you are giving the patient. *(True or False?)*

SHORT ANSWER QUESTIONS

1 In your own words, provide a definition of cultural competence.

2 In a few sentences, describe how your cultural background may differ from that of a patient or colleague. What are some of the cultural biases you have experienced or witnessed?

3 List at least three forms of nonverbal communication the HCP should be aware of when working with patients of different cultures.

4 Briefly describe at least two ways in which smiling can be interpreted in different cultures.

CLINICAL APPLICATIONS

1 Interview at least three people from cultures other than your own and ask them if they have ever encountered any communication problems with an HCP that resulted from cultural differences. Discuss

specifically what the sources of these problems were. How as an HCP would you approach these situations differently?

2 In the examination room waiting for you and your medical interpreter is a 63-year-old female patient from Japan. She has come into the medical practice because of a bad case of psoriasis that has developed recently. In order to treat her, you will need to examine her scalp. What should you tell the interpreter before you enter the room? What are some of the possible sources of misunderstanding that you anticipate before entering?

3 Find photographs from magazines that you believe show the following facial expressions: (a) happiness, (b) sadness, (c) fear, (d) anger, (e) disgust, and (f) surprise. Show these photos to friends or classmates from different cultures without telling them what emotions you have assigned to the photos. Ask your friends or classmates to interpret the emotions in the photos. Discuss any differences in interpretation.

Fundamental Writing Skills

The section in the writing skills chapter you should complete at the end of Chapter 8 is Section 10-8. You can find this section on pages 233–235.

SUGGESTED FURTHER READING

1. Axtell RE. *Gestures: The Do's and Taboos of Body Language around the World*. New York: Wiley; 1998.
2. Balzer Riley J. *Communication in Nursing*. 6th Ed. St. Louis: Mosby; 2007.
3. Betancourt JR, Like RC. Editorial: A new framework of care. *Patient Care. Special Issue, Caring for Diverse Populations: Breaking Down Barriers*, May 15, 2000:10–12.
4. Brach C, Fraser I. Can cultural competency reduce racial and ethnic health disparities? A review and conceptual model. *Med Care Res Rev*. 2000; 57(Suppl. 1):181–217.
5. Campinha-Bacote J. A model and instrument for addressing cultural competence in health care. *J Nurs Educ*. 1999;38(5):203–207.
6. Campinha-Bacote J. The Process of Cultural Competence in the Delivery of Healthcare Services (website). 2007. Retrieved May 2010 from http://www. transculturalcare.net/Cultural_Competence_Model.htm.
7. Cassey MZ. Using technology to support the CLAS standards. *Nurs Econ*. 2008;26(2):133–135.
8. Coombs G, Sarason Y. Culture circles: A cultural self-awareness exercise. *J Manage Educ*. 1998;22(2):218–226. Accessed May 25, 2010, from ABI/ INFORM Global.

9. Dixon LD. A case study of an intercultural health care visit: an African American woman and her white male physician. *Women and Language.* 2004;27(1):45–52.

10. Dresser N. *Multicultural Manners: New Rules of Etiquette for a Changing Society.* New York: Wiley; 1996.

11. Ferguson WJ, Candib LM. Culture, language, and the doctor-patient relationship. *Fam Med.* 2002;34(5):353–361.

12. Fleming M, Towey K. *Delivering Culturally Effective Health Care to Adolescents.* Chicago: American Medical Association; 2003.

13. Galambos CM. Moving cultural diversity toward cultural competence in health care. *Health Soc Work.* 2003;28(1):3–7.

14. Goode TD. *The Cultural Competence Continuum.* The National Center for Cultural Competence. Georgetown University Center for Child and Human Development, University Center for Excellence in Developmental Disabilities. Revised 2004. Retrieved May 22, 2010 from http://gucchd.georgetown. edu/nccc.

15. Harris SM, Majors R. Cultural value differences: implications for the experiences of African-American men. *Jour of Men's Studies.* 1993;1(3):227.

16. Harvey AR, Rauch JB. A comprehensive Afrocentric rites of passage program for black male adolescents. *Health Soc Work.* 1997;22(1):30–37.

17. Henry J. Kaiser Family Foundation. "Eliminating Racial/Ethnic Disparities in Health Care: What are the Options?" October 24, 2008. Retrieved May 22, 2010 from http://www.kff.org/minorityhealth/h08_7830.cfm.

18. Hershberger PJ, Righter EL, Zryd TW, et al. Implementation of a process-oriented cultural proficiency curriculum. *J Health Care Poor Underserved.* 2008;19(2):478–483.

19. Kardong-Edgren S, Campinha-Bacote J. Cultural competency of graduating US Bachelor of Science nursing students. *Contemp Nurse.* 2008;28(1–2):37–44.

20. Kreier R. Crossing the cultural divide. *Am Med News.* 1999;42.4:12–14.

21. Ludwick R, and Silva MC. "Nursing Around the World: Cultural Values and Ethical Conflicts." *Online Journal of Issues in Nursing.* August 14, 2000. Available at: www.nursingworld.org. Accessed May 22, 2009.

22. McNeil, Jr. D. "U.S. Apologizes for Syphilis Tests in Guatemala." *The New York Times.* October 1, 2010. A1, A6.

23. The Office of Minority Health. U.S. Department of Health and Human Services. *National Standards on Culturally and Linguistically Appropriate Services*

24. *(CLAS).* 04/12/2007. Retrieved May 22, 2010 from http://www.omhrc.gov/templates/browse.aspx?lvl=2&lvlID=15.

25. "An Older and More Diverse Nation by Mid-Century." U. S. Census Bureau Publication CB08-123. Retrieved May 2010 from http://www.census.gov/newsroom/releases/archives/population/cb08-123.html.

26. Poole DL. Politically correct or culturally competent? *Health Soc Work.* 1998;23(3):163–166.

27. Salimbine S. *What Language Does Your Patient Hurt In: A Practical Guide to Culturally Competent Patient Care.* 2nd ed. St. Paul, MN: EMCParadigm: 2005.

28. Samovar LA, Porter RE, McDaniel ER. *Communication Between Cultures.* 6th ed. Belmont, CA: Thomson; 2007.

29. Schulman KA, Berlin J, Harless W, et al. The effect of race and sex on physicians' recommendations for cardiac catheterization. *N Engl J Med.* 1999; 340(8):618–626.

30. Smedley BD, Stith AY, Nelson AR, eds. *Committee on Understanding and Eliminating Racial and Ethnic Disparities in Health Care.* Board on Health Sciences Policy, Institute of Medicine; 2003.

31. Smedley BD, Stith AY, Nelson AR, eds. *Unequal Treatment: Confronting Racial and Ethnic Disparities in Health Care.* Washington DC: The National Academies Press; 2003.

32. Taylor O. *Cross Cultural Communication—an Essential Dimension of Effective Education.* Chevy Chase, MD: The Mid-Atlantic Equity Center; 1987.

33. Taylor-Brown S, Garcia A, Kingson E. Cultural competence versus cultural chauvinism: Implications for social work. *Health Soc Work.* 2001;26(3): 185–187.

34. "Tripling of Hispanic and Asian Populations in 50 Years; Non-Hispanic Whites May Drop to Half of Total Population." U.S. Census Bureau publication CB04-44. Retrieved December 2009 from http://www.census.gov/Press-Release/www/releases/archives/population/001720.html.

35. "U.S. Interim Projections by Age, Sex, Race, and Hispanic Origin: 2000-2050." U.S. Census Bureau. Retrieved May 2010 from http://www.census.gov/population/www/projections/usinterimproj/.

36. Wilson-Stronks A, Lee KK, Cordero CL, et al. *One Size Does Not Fit All: Meeting the Health Care Needs of Diverse Populations.* Oakbrook Terrace, IL: The Joint Commission; 2008.

37. Wilson-Stronks A, Galvez E. *Hospitals, Language, and Culture: A Snap shot of the Nation Findings from a National Study of 60 Hospitals.* Oakbrook Terrace, IL: The Joint Commission; 2007.

Part III

ADMINISTRATIVE COMMUNICATION SKILLS

9

ELECTRONIC COMMUNICATION

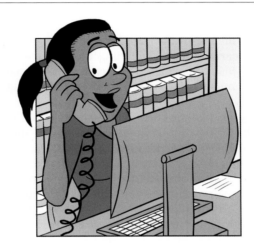

OBJECTIVES

- Explain how telecommunication, facsimile (fax), and email differ from face-to-face communication
- Discuss the guidelines for the effective use of the telephone in the healthcare setting
- Identify the types of incoming patient calls that are commonly handled by healthcare professionals
- Discuss the guidelines for dealing effectively with an angry patient
- Describe the minimum information needed for a telephone message taken in a healthcare setting
- Identify the types of incoming nonpatient calls that are commonly handled by healthcare professionals
- Define telephone triage and explain why it is an important procedure
- Discuss the guidelines for effectively handling potential emergency calls
- List the symptoms and conditions that require immediate medical help

■ Describe the type of information an emergency dispatcher will require and its significance
■ List the items of information that should be included on a facsimile (fax) cover sheet
■ Discuss the guidelines for the secure operation of a facsimile (fax) machine
■ Discuss the guidelines for the effective use of email in the healthcare setting

There are several means for the transfer of incoming and outgoing information in healthcare settings, including face-to-face discussion, telephone, facsimile (fax), and email. Healthcare professionals (HCPs) must be able to communicate efficiently and effectively using each of these forms.

The majority of this book has addressed face-to-face communication, in which the HCP and the patient communicate directly with each other. This is clearly the most effective form of interaction between individuals, as 100% of a message may be imparted by the sender (7% verbal communication, 23% tone of voice, 70% nonverbal communication). Furthermore, the receiver of the message can ask for clarification if necessary. Face-to-face communication is the best method for delivering the maximum amount of information in a message. However, for many reasons, such as time constraints and distance, it is not always the most practical method. Therefore, other methods may be employed to transfer information.

Telecommunication, or the use of a telephone, is one of the most important forms of communication between HCPs and their patients as well as their colleagues. However, only 30% of a message may be imparted by the sender (7% verbal, 23% tone of voice). The majority of the message (70%), the nonverbal portion of the message such as eye contact, facial expression and posture, cannot be observed over the telephone. The advantage of this form of communication is that it allows for immediate interaction between the sender and the receiver of the message. During the telephone conversation, the receiver of the message can ask questions for clarification and the sender can provide a direct response.

Written communication in the healthcare setting may include facsimile and email. This is a very practical method for the transmission of medical records, physician's orders, and test results from one HCP to another. However, a disadvantage of this form of communication is that only 7% of the message, the words chosen by the sender, is available for interpretation by the receiver. Both tone of voice and the nonverbal portion of the message are unavailable to the receiver. Furthermore, the

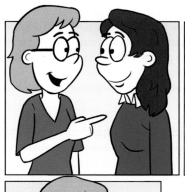
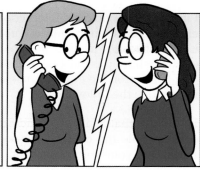

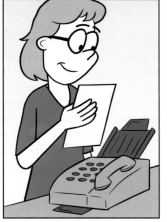

FIGURE 9-1. Modalities of Communication.
(A) Face-to-face communication is the most effective form of interaction between individuals as 100% of the message (verbal communication, tone of voice, and nonverbal communication) is available for interpretation by the receiver. **(B)** When communicating on the telephone, only 30% of the message may be imparted by the sender (verbal communication and tone of voice.) **(C)** Written communication allows only approximately 7% of the message (verbal communication) to be available for interpretation by the receiver.

written form of communication does not allow for immediate interaction between the sender and the receiver as the receiver cannot have their questions answered instantly.

This chapter focuses on the appropriate and effective use of the telephone by HCPs in the clinical setting. The discussion includes various types of incoming calls, methods of handling calls from angry patients, telephone triage, and instructions for making emergency calls. The proper use of facsimile machines and email is also addressed.

Telecommunication

Telephone Etiquette

As the person who answers the telephone, you are the representative of your medical office or department. In fact, you may be the first impression that a patient or medical colleague has of your particular clinical setting. Consider how many "relationships" you may have with people you have never met. Proper telephone etiquette, or good manners, is vital in ensuring a positive interaction between people communicating by telephone. This is particularly true in many healthcare settings where additional obstacles such as possible patient distress and surrounding noise and distractions must be overcome.

Guidelines for the effective use of the telephone in the healthcare setting include the following:

- Use a voice that is pleasant and professional. Speak directly into the receiver. Hold the mouthpiece one to two inches from your mouth and project your voice toward it. Use a normal conversational tone and speak at a natural pace. Pronounce words correctly to avoid misunderstandings. Finally, good enunciation, or clear, distinct speaking, will help the caller to understand you.
- Use proper inflection. In other words, alter the pitch and tone of your voice. This will prevent a droning, monotonous speaking style, which may be interpreted as boredom or lack of caring.
- Be courteous. Speak to the caller politely, even if you have been interrupted or if you are in a stressful environment such as an emergency room. Avoid sounding impatient or irritated. Instead, be friendly, smile, and project a caring, helpful attitude. It may sound silly, but the caller really can "hear" your smile as it affects your tone of voice. Use tact and sensitivity. Finally, use the person's name and thank the caller before ending the conversation.
- Give the caller your undivided attention. In a busy clinical setting, it may be tempting to try to multitask or continue with other activities while speaking on the telephone. This activity is likely to lead to errors in documentation or an inaccurate understanding of the message being conveyed by the caller. The best practice is to give the caller the same undivided attention that you would give to a person in front of you.
- Paraphrase to ensure accurate understanding of the caller's message.
- Never answer the telephone and immediately place the caller on hold. Instead, ask the caller if they would mind holding and wait for an answer. Be sure that the call is not an emergency before placing the caller on hold.
- Identify the caller. When you receive a call from a person who claims to be a patient, take steps to identify the caller. In this way, patient confidentiality is protected. Depending upon your office or department, forms of identifying information that may be requested include the patient's first and last names, social security number, date of birth, and address. You may verify this information using the patient's computer record or their medical chart.
- Do not repeat confidential information over the telephone if patients or other unauthorized people are within hearing distance. As with

caller identification, this will also assist in maintaining patient confidentiality.

■ Let the caller hang up first. Before hanging up, be sure that the conversation has been adequately completed. This will increase the likelihood that the caller feels properly cared for and satisfied. Allowing the caller to hang up first will assist in avoiding an abrupt end to the conversation.

Types of Incoming Calls

A doctor's office or the nurse's desk in a hospital or nursing home will receive many different types of calls over the course of the day (and even night). The caller must be treated with the same courtesy and respect as a patient who is physically present. Attempt to answer the call by the second ring. Identify yourself and your office or department and offer your assistance. Examples of both patient calls and nonpatient calls are discussed below.

Patient Calls

Appointments
Appointment requests are one of the most common types of calls to a doctor's office or medical department. Follow office policy for routine patient visits. Other requests may involve patients with health problems. In this case, follow telephone triage procedures (discussed in the next section) to schedule the appointment appropriately.

Billing Inquiries
Health insurance in the United States has become increasingly complex. For example, the multitude of different private insurance companies, state insurance providers, and federal insurance providers (Medicaid and Medicare) all have different policies and benefits. There are differences in copayments, deductibles, and coinsurance. Some medical procedures are covered by a certain insurance provider and others are not. A given clinician may not accept a particular type of insurance. Many patients do not have a thorough understanding of their specific health insurance. As a result, patients will often call with the question "Why did I receive this bill?" or "Why was this appointment or procedure not fully covered?" As an HCP, you will need to answer these questions courteously and accurately. If the patient remains dissatisfied, document all relevant comments and report the conversation to the office or department manager.

Diagnostic Test Results
Many laboratory and radiology reports are called in to the physician's office before the written report is sent to the patient. The HCP must

follow office policy regarding the dissemination of these results. In some offices, the HCP may be authorized to report favorable (normal or negative) test results to the patient by telephone. Abnormal or unsatisfactory test results are reported to the patient by the physician.

Medication Inquiries

Patients may call with questions about their current prescriptions. These inquiries may involve how to take the medication properly as well as potential side effects. Patients may also desire information regarding new medications and the possibility that a drug may be beneficial for their condition. These calls must be referred to the physician, physician assistant, or nurse practitioner in the practice.

Requests for Advice

Occasionally, a patient will call a medical office or hospital emergency room and ask for advice regarding their condition. HCPs are not trained to make a diagnosis, prescribe a medication, or give medical advice of any kind. Politely tell the patient that they must see the physician or other qualified healthcare provider. If the patient cannot come to the office, assure the patient that the physician will return their call or advise them to visit an emergency room.

ROLE **PLAY** | **Types of Incoming Patient Calls**

In groups of three to four—one patient caller, one HCP, and one to two observers—take turns playing the patient and the HCP and acting out the following scenarios. Apply the guidelines for proper telephone etiquette.

1 A 28-year-old man calls the doctor's office to make an appointment for his persistent rash.
2 A 19-year-old female college student has never had to worry about healthcare insurance or paying healthcare bills before. She wants to know why she has received a bill for $20 for a recent appointment with a gynecologist.
3 A 45-year-old woman calls the doctor's office and identifies herself as her 23-year-old daughter. Although she does not know her daughter's social security number, she wants to know the results of her daughter's pregnancy test.
4 A 67-year-old man calls the doctor's office to report that he is feeling light-headed and dizzy. He recently began taking a diuretic for his high blood pressure and he wants to know if the medication might be responsible for his symptoms.

Discuss what was effective in facilitating communication with the patient. What impaired communication?

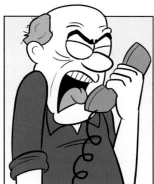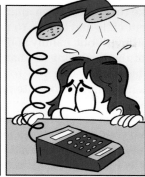

FIGURE 9-2. The Angry Patient. The most important thing to remember when handling a call from an angry patient is not to lose your own temper. Remain calm and empathic. Try to calm the patient and assure them that you want to help.

The Angry Patient

Even when a medical office or department delivers the best care possible, there will still be calls from angry or upset patients. The most important thing to remember when handling a call from an angry patient is not to lose your own temper. Remain mindful that although some patients may simply be angry about waiting on hold, other patients are often displacing their apparent anger and are most likely frustrated with worry about illness or suffering from pain. The best approach is to be empathic while remaining in control of the situation. Try to calm the patient and assure them that you want to help. Guidelines for dealing with an angry patient include the following:

- Listen carefully and acknowledge the patient's anger.
- Do not interrupt the patient.
- Remain calm. Speak gently and kindly to the patient. Assure the patient that you care and that you want to help them.
- Avoid talking down to the patient or appearing to be condescending as this is likely to make the situation worse.
- Do not place blame on the patient.
- Avoid becoming defensive.
- Never make promises that cannot be kept.
- Take careful notes and be sure to document the call. Include the problem and the outcome. Inform the appropriate physician or supervisor even after the problem has been resolved.
- Inform the appropriate physician or supervisor if the patient threatens legal action against the office, hospital, or clinic.
- If it is necessary to consult with another person regarding the patient's problem, be sure to inform the patient as to when they may

expect to hear from you. Anxiously waiting for the telephone to ring may make the patient even angrier.

■ If a patient calls and begins to rant and rave about an issue that you know nothing about, calmly and in a soft tone of voice, ask the patient to start at the beginning so that you may fully understand their concerns. This will enable you to either assist the patient yourself or direct them to the appropriate person or department that can resolve their problem.

■ If the patient is speaking so loudly that you must hold the receiver away from your ear, ask the caller to hold for just a moment while you obtain their chart. This interlude may allow the patient to calm down.

■ If the patient uses profanity, remind the patient that you are there to help them but cannot continue the call unless you are spoken to in a courteous manner. It may be necessary to transfer the call to your supervisor or office manager.

| ROLE |
| **PLAY** |

The Angry Patient

In groups of three to four—one patient caller, one HCP, and one to two observers—take turns playing the patient and the HCP and acting out the following scenarios. Apply the guidelines for effectively handling an angry patient.

1 **A 50-year-old man receives a telephone message stating that his colonoscopy has been rescheduled for the second time due to other medical emergencies. Because he is anxious about the procedure, he is very upset when he calls the doctor's office to complain about the rescheduling.**

2 **A 27-year-old woman is prescribed a medication for the first time. She is counseled that a potential side effect of the drug is nausea and vomiting. After taking two doses, she becomes nauseous and vomits several times. When she calls the doctor's office, she screams at the HCP about how angry she is that the doctor has prescribed this horrible medication.**

Discuss what was effective in facilitating communication with the patient. What impaired communication?

Nonpatient Calls

Family Members or Friends of a Patient
The nurse's desk in a hospital or nursing home will often receive calls regarding a patient from concerned family members or friends of the patient. Remember that a patient's medical information is confidential. Health Insurance Portability and Accountability Act (HIPAA) standards

require that the patient provide their authorization prior to the release of their information (Chapter 4).

Other Physicians, Hospital Departments, or Healthcare Facilities

Patients typically receive care from a team of providers including the primary physician, physician specialists, nurses, and a wide variety of allied health professionals. As mentioned previously, an efficient method of communication between these individuals is the use of the telephone. Consulting about patient care, reporting test results, conveying orders for treatment, and scheduling are just a few of the topics of conversation between members of the healthcare team. Office or departmental policies, professionalism, and patient confidentiality must all be considered when speaking with other healthcare colleagues about a shared patient.

Prescription Refill Requests

Other common incoming calls to a doctor's office are requests for prescription refills. Many offices have a voice mail system and a set of office policies for handling these requests. These calls may originate from a patient or a pharmacy.

The Telephone Message

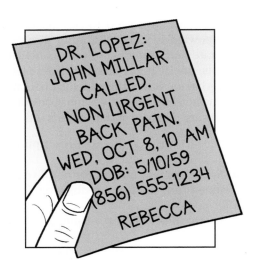

FIGURE 9-3. The telephone message.

In any healthcare setting, a call may come in for someone who is not available. In this case, the receiver of the call must take a telephone message. The minimum information needed for a message includes the following:

- First and last name of the caller
- Relationship to the patient
- Patient's date of birth
- Date and time of the call
- Telephone number where the caller can be reached (Always verify the callback number. The lack of a return call due to an incorrect number may be misinterpreted as a lack of concern or respect.)
- Brief description of the reason for the call
- Urgency of the call
- Name of the person the caller is trying to reach
- Name or initials of the person taking the message

If possible, after you have taken the message, tell the caller when they are likely to expect a return call.

Telephone Triage

The term *triage* refers to the screening and sorting of emergency incidents. In other words, triage is the process used to determine the order of priority or urgency with which patients should be treated. Because a medical practice typically has multiple telephone lines, the allied health professional may receive several patient calls at the same time and, accordingly, have to determine the order in which to handle them. Once again, use of the telephone prevents visual inspection of the patient or face-to-face interaction. Therefore, the HCP will need to rely on their communication skills and their knowledge of health and disease processes in order to obtain an accurate understanding of each patient's symptoms or concerns. In other words, the HCP must have excellent listening skills to be aware of the nonverbal messages the patients are conveying regarding pain, anxiety, fear, and level of comprehension. Consider the instance in which four patient calls are received at the doctor's office.

- Line 1: A pharmacy technician wants to verify a patient's prescription refill.
- Line 2: A new mother wants to make an appointment for her 3-year-old daughter who has a fever (temperature 100.2° Fahrenheit, or 37.8° Celsius).
- Line 3: A very anxious caller is trying to get his test results and has been accidentally disconnected twice.
- Line 4: An 88-year-old woman having chest pain wonders whether the doctor might have any time to see her.

Which of these calls should be prioritized and handled first? Why? Which call is the least urgent and should be handled last? Why? To effectively process these calls, the HCP must be able to distinguish routine incoming calls from urgent calls. Furthermore, they must be able to distinguish panicked or hysterical callers from true medical emergencies. Guidelines for handling potential emergency calls include the following:

- Remain calm: This demeanor will help to soothe the caller so that you may be able to obtain the necessary information efficiently.
- Obtain the following information:
    - Caller's name, telephone number, and the address from which they are making the call; in case you are disconnected, you may immediately return the call or, if necessary, send an ambulance.
    - Caller's relationship to the patient
    - Patient's name, age, and date of birth
    - Nature of the emergency: What happened? When did it happen? Where did it happen? How severe is it?
    - If the caller is the patient, determine whether there is anyone else present
    - Complete description of the patient's symptoms and how they are reacting to the situation
    - Any treatment that has been administered to the patient
    - Whether an ambulance has been called
    - Name of the patient's primary care physician
- If the situation is indeed a medical emergency, put the call through to the physician immediately.
- If the situation is not a medical emergency, handle the call according to office or departmental policies.
- If there is any doubt, treat the call as a medical emergency. It is better to err on the side of caution. The physician or other qualified medical personnel should make the decision.

Symptoms and conditions require that immediate medical help are found in Table 9-1. With these criteria, let us reconsider the four patient calls that were received at the doctor's office.

- Line 4: This caller should be taken first. Her chest pain may be a sign of a life-threatening situation, such as a heart attack, and is the top priority.
- Line 3: The caller on Line 3 should be taken second. Although it is not an emergency, the patient is already upset. The longer he waits, the more upset he may become and the more difficult he may be to please.
- Line 2: This caller should be taken third. Although not currently life-threatening, a fever of this magnitude has the potential to become serious. Make an appointment for the mother and her daughter for as soon as possible.
- Line 1: The caller on Line 1 should be taken last as this is a routine call with no urgency whatsoever.

TABLE 9-1

Symptoms and Conditions that Require Immediate Medical Help

- Symptoms of a heart attack: chest pain; pain radiating to the arm, neck, or shoulder; sweating; weakness; pallor
- Symptoms of a stroke: slurred speech, sudden inability to move a body part or one side of the body, seizures, severe headache
- Allergic reactions to drugs, food, or insect stings: symptoms include difficulty breathing, vomiting, pallor, and weak and rapid pulse
- Symptoms of heatstroke: flushed skin that is hot; a strong and rapid pulse, confusion, or loss of consciousness
- Premature labor
- Suicide attempt or suicide threat
- Severe pain of any kind
- Difficulty breathing
- Asthmatic attack
- Profuse bleeding
- Loss of consciousness
- Severe vomiting
- Severe diarrhea
- Fever with temperature greater than 102° Fahrenheit, or 38.8° Celsius
- Broken bones

ROLE **PLAY**   **The Medical Emergency**

In groups of three to four—one patient caller, one HCP, and one to two observers—take turns playing the patient and the HCP and acting out the following scenarios. Apply the guidelines for effectively handling a medical emergency.

1 **A 23-year-old man has severe abdominal pain and a fever (temperature 102.6° Fahrenheit, or 39.2° Celsius). He calls the doctor's office to see if they think it is serious.**
2 **It is the height of the allergy season. A 30-year-old woman who is not asthmatic experiences mild wheezing. She calls the doctor's office in a panic regarding this symptom.**

Discuss what was effective in facilitating communication with the patient. What impaired communication?

Outgoing Emergency Calls

On occasion, a patient may need immediate assistance that can only be provided in a hospital emergency room. For example, consider the instance where a patient appears to have a heart attack in a doctor's office or a nursing home. The responding doctors and R.N.'s will be occupied providing lifesaving procedures to the patient. As the associated allied health professional (e.g., medical assistant, C.N.A.), you will need to call for an ambulance and the emergency medical technicians (EMTs) by dialing 911. The responding 911 dispatcher will ask for the following information:

- Patient's name, age, and gender: Age is of particular importance when the patient is an infant or small child.
- Nature of the medical problem (e.g., chest pain, apparent stroke, severe abdominal pain, bleeding)
- Level of service requested by the physician: Emergency responders may provide either basic life support or advanced life support.
- Specific instructions or requests from the physician: Typically, the ambulance will transport the patient to the nearest hospital. However, the patient's condition or diagnosis may necessitate an alternative destination. For example, an infant or child may be sent to a children's hospital instead of a community hospital.
- Location of the emergency and any specific instructions for access (e.g., Milton Nursing Home, 570 Brush Hill Road, second floor, room 221)

Speak to the dispatcher in a slow, calm voice. Ask the dispatcher for an approximate time of arrival for the ambulance. Report this information to the clinicians treating the patient. Do not end the call until instructed to do so by the dispatcher.

ROLE **PLAY** **Outgoing Emergency Calls**

In groups of three to four—one 911-dispatcher, one HCP, and one to two observers—take turns playing the dispatcher and the HCP and acting out the following scenarios. Apply the guidelines for effectively handling an outgoing emergency call.

1 **A 74-year-old woman knits while waiting to see her cardiologist. A medical assistant looks out into the waiting room to see that the woman has stopped knitting, her face is drooped on the right side and her right arm rests in her lap. When the medical assistant alerts the cardiologist, they instruct her to immediately call 911.**

2 **A 92-year-old man is in his wheelchair in the sunroom of his nursing home. He suddenly clutches his chest and appears to be in severe pain. A passing C.N.A. notices him and alerts the nurse on duty. The C.N.A. then calls for an ambulance.**

Discuss what was effective in facilitating communication with the 911 dispatcher. What impaired communication?

Facsimile, or Fax

Facsimile, or fax, machines, send and receive printed materials over a telephone line. Faxes provide an easy, quick, and cost-effective method of transferring information. This method may be used to transmit medical records, physician's orders, and test results.

The first page to be faxed is always the cover sheet. The following information should be included on this sheet:

■ Name, address, telephone number, and fax number of the office or department to which the fax is being sent
■ Name of the healthcare professional for whom the fax is intended
■ Date and time of the fax
■ Number of pages transmitted (including the cover sheet)
■ Confidentiality statement

The confidentiality statement is necessary because the content of the fax may be private. Any fax containing patient information is protected by HIPAA privacy rules. Accordingly, a potential disadvantage to sending confidential information via fax machine is the lack of confidentiality. If the receiving machine is occupied with incoming or outgoing faxes, then the sending machine will continue to automatically redial the number until it can send the fax. As a result, unauthorized individuals may have access to the transmitted document. Guidelines for the secure operation of a fax machine include the following:

■ Inform the recipient of your outgoing document prior to faxing confidential information so that they may immediately retrieve it.
■ Immediately remove your incoming faxes from the machine.
■ Place fax machines in a secure location to minimize the possibility of unauthorized access to faxes.

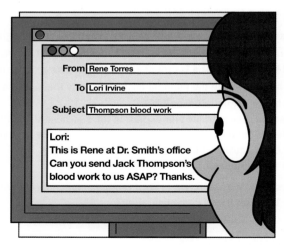

FIGURE 9-4. Email. The use of email is an efficient method of communication between HCPs.

Email

Email is an almost instantaneous and essentially cost-free method of transmitting written information. It is faster and more spontaneous than a letter sent by the U.S. Postal Service; however, email is permanent like a posted letter. This may be of concern when there is a disagreement between the individuals involved.

Email messages are most effective when they are short and to the point. However, it is important to be mindful that these messages can seem very cold. When emailing a patient, the HCP must make an effort to compose a message that appears warm and caring.

Email may also be used to send longer documents as attachments. Be sure to open the document before sending the email to confirm that the correct document is attached.

Guidelines for the effective use of email in the healthcare setting include the following:

- Use the subject line to inform the recipient about the content of the email.
- Prepare an email with a message and a format that is appropriate for the intended recipient. Emails to physicians, supervisors, or individuals with whom you are not acquainted may require a higher degree of formality than emails sent to colleagues with whom you have a more casual relationship. Include a greeting such as Dear Dr. Roberts. Use complete sentences with correct capitalization. Check the spelling. Finally, sign the message and provide your contact information.
- Do not use all capital, or uppercase, letters. This may be interpreted as shouting.
- Avoid sending confidential messages via email without prior agreement by both the sender and the receiver. Families may share an email account, which could allow another member to read your patient's message.
- Include a confidentiality statement at the end of the email similar to that on the fax cover sheet.

REVIEW QUESTIONS

OBJECTIVE QUESTIONS

1 The system of prioritizing patient telephone calls according to the degree of urgency is referred to as _____.
2 When a patient calls for medical advice, it is better for the HCP to provide the information directly to the patient to avoid interrupting the doctor. *(True or false?)*

3 When unsure as to whether a caller has an actual medical emergency, it is better for the HCP to assume that it is, in fact, an emergency and alert the physician. *(True or false?)*
4 Fax cover sheets and emails originating from a healthcare facility should contain a confidentiality statement. *(True or false?)*
5 Emails to other healthcare providers should be written using all capital, or uppercase, letters so that they are easier to read quickly. *(True or false?)*
6 Abnormal or unsatisfactory test results should be reported to the patient on the telephone only by the physician. *(True or false?)*

SHORT ANSWER QUESTIONS

1 Describe five communication skills that are used when speaking on a telephone. Include how these skills contribute to effective communication.
2 List five symptoms or conditions that require immediate medical attention.
3 Define telephone triage. Provide examples of four different incoming telephone calls and how you would triage each call.
4 Explain how telecommunication, fax, and email differ from face-to-face communication.
5 Discuss two factors that enhance the secure operation of a fax machine.
6 Discuss three factors that contribute to the effective use of email.

CLINICAL APPLICATION

1 Mrs. Ryan is a 77-year-old woman with stomach cancer. Following surgery, she continued treatment with chemotherapy. When it was discovered that the cancer had spread to her liver and her bones, she elected to discontinue the chemotherapy and began palliative care, which does not fight the cancer but keeps a patient as comfortable as possible. Upon learning of her decision, her 50-year-old son Joseph became distraught and called the oncologist's office demanding that he speak with the doctor immediately. Danielle is a medical assistant who answered Joseph's call. She explained that the doctor takes only emergency calls during appointment hours but that she will take a detailed message. Joseph insists that this is indeed an emergency and that if he is not put through to the doctor, he will sue the doctor for malpractice regarding his mother.
   ■ Should this call be treated as an emergency and receive top priority? Why or why not?

- What should Danielle do to placate this angry caller?
- How could Danielle unintentionally make the situation worse?
- What patient confidentiality issues should be considered with this caller?
- If Joseph agrees to leave a message, what information should Danielle obtain?

2 Maura is a 26-year-old pregnant woman who is waiting to see her gynecologist. When she gets up to get a new magazine, she realizes that she has been bleeding profusely. Jane, the medical assistant, immediately alerts the doctor who reaches Maura as she begins to faint. As the doctor attends to Maura, Jane calls for an ambulance.

- Why did Jane call for an ambulance?
- What information did she provide to the 911 dispatcher?
- What information did she obtain from the 911 dispatcher?
- What telecommunication skills could Maura employ to facilitate her interaction with the 911 dispatcher?

Fundamental Writing Skills

The section in the writing skills chapter you should complete at the end of Chapter 9 is Section 10-9. You can find this section on pages 235–236.

SUGGESTED FURTHER READING

1. American Red Cross. *Nurse Assistant Training*. Yardley, PA: Staywell; 2002.
2. Beaman N, Fleming-McPhillips L. *Pearson's Comprehensive Medical Assisting, Administrative and Clinical Competencies*. Upper Saddle River, NJ: Pearson Prentice Hall; 2007.
3. Booth KA, Whicker LG, Wyman TD, et al. *Medical Assisting, Administrative and Clinical Procedures Including Anatomy & Physiology*. 3rd ed. New York: McGraw Hill; 2009.
4. Colbert BJ. *Workplace Readiness for Health Occupations*. New York: Delmar Publishers; 2000.
5. Courson S. What is telephone nurse triage? *Connections Magazine*, Retrieved May 2010, from http://www.connectionsmagazine.com/articles/5/090.html.
6. Drafke MW. *Working in Health Care, What You Need to Know to Succeed*. 2nd ed. Philadelphia: F.A. Davis; 2002.
7. Kale-Smith G. *Medical Assisting Made Incredibly Easy, Administrative Competencies*. Philadelphia: Lippincott Williams & Wilkins; 2008.
8. Keir L, Wise BA, Krebs C. *Medical Assisting, Administrative and Clinical Competencies*. 5th ed. Clifton Park, NY: Thomson Delmar Learning; 2003.

9. Lindh WQ, Pooler MS, Tamparo CD, et al. *Comprehensive Medical Assisting, Administrative and Clinical Competencies.* 3rd ed. Clifton Park, NY: Thomson Delmar Learning; 2006.

10. Molle EA, Kronenberger J, Durham LS, et al. *Lippincott William & Wilkins' Comprehensive Medical Assisting.* 2nd ed. Philadelphia: Lippincott Williams & Wilkins; 2005.

11. Riley JB. *Communication in Nursing.* 6th ed. St. Louis: Mosby Elsevier; 2008.

12. Sanderson SM. *Case Studies for the Medical Office, Capstone Billing Simulation.* 5th ed. New York: McGraw Hill; 2010.

13. U. S. Department of Health & Human Services. Can a physician's office FAX patient medical information to another physician's office? Retrieved May 2010 from http://www.hhs.gov/hipaafaq/use/356.html.

10

FUNDAMENTAL WRITING SKILLS

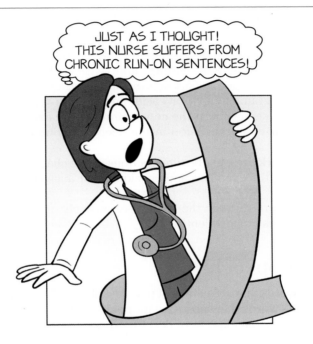

OBJECTIVES

- Explain the functions and purposes of the parts of speech and punctuation
- Illustrate correct sentence grammar
- Identify common sentence errors and strategies for correcting them
- Demonstrate effective paragraph basics
- Explain the basics of SOAP notes

Section 10-1 (To accompany Chapter 1, "The Communication Process")

This chapter provides a basic guide to the essentials of grammar. Grammar is the foundation upon which all good writing rests. Grammar matters.

Although we cannot promise that having an understanding of grammar alone will make you a better writer, we can say with confidence that without an understanding of grammar, you will have a much harder time becoming a good writer. Good writing skills are important in all of the healthcare professions. You will find that the further you advance in your healthcare career, the more you will have to write. The more you have to write, the stronger your writing skills need to be.

This chapter provides a thorough review of grammar, a basic overview of effective paragraph construction, and a brief introduction to SOAP (Subjective-Objective-Assessment-Plan) note taking. You can use the chapter in one of three ways.

1 You can work through the chapter one section at a time, completing one of the nine sections along with each of the first nine chapters of the book. This step-by-step method will make completing the grammar section easier and less burdensome over the course of a semester. At the conclusion of each exercise, you can check your comprehension in the accompanying online answer key.

2 You can work through the nine sections of the chapter in sequence, completing the exercises and checking your answers in the online key.

3 You can work through the chapter exclusively online, completing the exercises independently.

Parts of Speech

- Nouns—words that are names of persons, places, things, or concepts
- Pronouns—words that substitute for nouns or refer to nouns
- Verbs—words that express or describe actions or states of being
- Adjectives—words that modify or describe nouns or pronouns
- Adverbs—words that modify or describe verbs, adjectives, or other adverbs
- Prepositions—words that show relationships of time or space
- Conjunctions—words that connect and show relationships between words, phrases, or clauses

Nouns

Nouns are words that are names of persons, places, things, or concepts. Examples of nouns are *stethoscope, patient, information, virus, bed.*

Countable Nouns
Countable nouns name things that you can count: *two nurses, one scale, five desks, six books.*

Noncountable Nouns
Noncountable nouns name things that you cannot count, so they cannot take plural forms: *information, advice, patience, knowledge.*

Proper Nouns
Proper nouns name particular people, places, organizations, months, days of the week, and they are always capitalized: *Dr. Jones, Boston, Glendale Memorial Hospital, January, Tuesday.*

Common Nouns
Common nouns name general persons, places, organizations, things or ideas: *doctor, city, hospital, month, day, treatment.*

Collective Nouns
Collective nouns name groups but are normally written in the singular form: *a committee, a healthcare team, a nursing pool, a faculty.*

| **PRACTICE WITH** **NOUNS** |

Identify the types of nouns in bold print as proper nouns (PN), common nouns (CN), or collective nouns (CO). Underline all noncountable nouns.

1 **John** has been a **member** of the college **faculty** since he arrived in **Baltimore**.
2 Dr. **Martin** has some **experience** with elderly **patients.**
3 Mrs. Murphy's **daughter** will accompany her during the **examination.**
4 I think you can find the **thermometer** in the **cabinet** above the **sink.**
5 The **information** in the **chart** is not accurate, according to Dr. **Benson.**

Pronouns

Pronouns are words that replace or refer to nouns or other pronouns. The noun or pronoun it replaces or refers to is called its *antecedent.*
   As examples, take the following sentences:

■ Dr. Rodriguez brought his stethoscope to work this morning.
   ■ *Dr. Rodriguez* is the antecedent of *his.*
■ Ms. Johnson brought her x-rays to the appointment with Dr. Rodriguez.
   ■ *Ms. Johnson* is the antecedent of *her.*
■ Ms. Johnson told Dr. Rodriguez that she had chest pains.
   ■ *Ms. Johnson* is the antecedent of *she.*

Personal Pronouns

Personal pronouns refer to particular people, places, or things. Personal pronouns have several different categories.

Box 10-1 Personal Pronouns

Subject Pronouns	Object Pronouns	Possessive Pronouns
I	me	my, mine
you	you	your, yours
he, she, it	him, her, it	his, her, hers, its
we	us	our, ours
they	them	their, theirs
who/whoever	whom/whomever	whose

Indefinite Pronouns

Indefinite pronouns do not refer to specific people, places, or things, and they do not need antecedents.

Box 10-2 Indefinite Pronouns

Singular	Plural	Singular or Plural
someone, somebody, something	both	all
anyone, anybody, anything	few	any
everyone, everybody, everything	many	most
no one, nobody, nothing	several	none
every, each		some

Relative Pronouns

Relative pronouns introduce dependent clauses (see Dependent Clauses later in this chapter): *who, whom, whoever, whomever, whichever, that, which.*

- Ms. Jones is the patient *who* has a pulmonary function test this morning.
- Genuineness and empathy are two of the many important qualities *that* a healthcare professional must possess.
- Dr. Rodriguez is the cardiologist *whom* Ms. Jones wants to see.

A note on the use of they: Throughout the text of this book, the authors have used the gender-neutral pronoun *they* when referring to any healthcare professional (HCP) or patient whose gender is not identified within the sentence where the pronoun appears. The authors have decided on this use of *they* – also called the singular, or epicene, *they* – to avoid the awkward repetition of such constructions as "his/her" or "his or her" that would appear in an instructional text of this kind in which examples of the interaction between an HCP and a patient must so frequently be used. Students should always remember to use the appropriate gender-specific pronoun he or she when the gender of the antecedent is clear.

| **PRACTICE WITH** | **PRONOUNS** |

Identify the pronouns in bold print by marking them as personal pronouns (PP), indefinite pronouns (IP), or relative pronouns (RP).

1 Mr. Henin is the patient **who** insists on bringing **his** dog with **him** to all appointments.
2 Is there **anyone** here **who** can tell me where Dr. Jett left **his** stethoscope?
3 I understand what **you** just told **me,** but **I** still insist that the book is **mine.**
4 Mr. Pierre gave the nurse **his** medical history without having **his** daughter there to remember everything for **him.**
5 Martha said **she** knows **someone** in dining services **who** can come up and speak with **my** mother.

Verbs

Verbs are words that express actions or states of being. Examples of verbs are *examine, study, treat, wash,* and *sterilize.*

Auxiliary Verbs

Auxiliary verbs are forms of *to be, to do,* and *to have* that help the main verb.

■ Dr. Pierre *was* examining Mr. North in Examination Room 3. (*to be: am, is, are, was, being, been*)
■ Susan Chang *does* make sure to get a complete history with every patient. (*to do: do, does, did*)
■ The x-rays *have* shown the scars on Mr. Frank's right lung. (*to have: have, has, had*)

Transitive Verbs
Transitive verbs show an action and transfer that action from the *subject* to a receiver, called a *direct object.*

■ The radiology technician examined the medical record. (*Technician* is the subject, *examined* is the transitive verb, and *record* is the direct object.)
■ The medical assistant took the patient's vital signs. (*Assistant* is the subject, *took* is the transitive verb, and *signs* is the direct object.)
■ The doctor is prescribing a new medication. (*Doctor* is the subject, *prescribing* is the transitive verb, and *medication* is the direct object.)
■ The nurse sees him. (*Nurse* is the subject, *sees* is the transitive verb, and *him* is the direct object.)

Intransitive Verbs

Intransitive verbs often show an action, but there is never a receiver of the action. Intransitive verbs can never take a direct object. Examples of intransitive verbs are sit, lie, sleep, die, breathe, and walk.

- The patient lies on the examination table. (The patient can lie *on* the examination table, but they cannot *lie* the examination table.)
- The medical assistant is sitting at the nursing station. (The medical assistant can sit *at* the nursing station, but they cannot *sit* the nursing station.)
- The nursing student slept through the night. (The nursing student can sleep *through* the night, but they cannot *sleep* the night.)

Linking Verbs

Linking verbs link a subject to a word after the verb. The word can be either an adjective or a noun that renames the subject. The most common linking verb is *to be* (am, is, are, was, were).

- Ms. Pontiac is asymptomatic. (*Asymptomatic* describes *Ms. Pontiac.*)
- Mr. Dodge was confused. (*Confused* describes Mr. Dodge.)
- Dr. Pound is a pulmonologist. (*Pulmonologist* renames *Dr. Pound.*)
- Jennifer is a radiology technologist. (*Radiology technologist* renames Jennifer.)

Other linking verbs can sometimes show a state of being. Examples of these are *feel, seem, look, taste, smell,* and *appear.*

- The medicine tastes bitter. (*Tastes* is the linking verb, and *bitter* describes the *medicine.*)
- The water looks clean. (*Looks* is the linking verb, and *clean* describes the *water.*)
- The child seems short of breath (*Seems* is the linking verb, and *short of breath* describes the *child.*)
- The nursing staff appears busy. (*Appears* is the linking verb, and *busy* describes the *staff.*)

The verb *to feel* can sometimes be a linking verb and sometimes a transitive verb. When you use the verb *to feel* to describe a person's emotional state, you use it as a linking verb. When you describe an action of the subject, you use it as a transitive verb.

- The nurses felt bad after the patient died. (*Bad* describes the *nurses' emotional state.*)
- The doctor felt the patient's underarms for any sign of swelling. (*Underarms* is the direct object of *felt.*)

PRACTICE WITH VERBS

Identify the verbs in bold print in the sentences below as transitive verbs (TV), intransitive verbs (IV), or linking verbs (LV).

1 The nutritionist **gave** the patient a brochure on diabetic diets.

2 The nurse **looked** sad after hearing that her former patient **had died.**

3 Dr. Jameson **felt** the patient's neck for swollen lymph nodes.

4 The medical assistant **called** the pharmacist with the new prescription.

5 Mrs. Benitez **drove** her car to the oncologist's office for the first round of chemotherapy.

6 The basketball coach **felt** bad when one of his players was injured in the game.

7 The patient **slept** quietly after the surgery.

8 Martin **watched** the instructional video on the proper method of taking a patient's blood pressure.

9 This wound **looks** infected.

10 The doctor **wrote** the prescription, but the pharmacist could not **read** it.

Verb Tenses

Verb tenses show the time of an action.

Box 10-3 Verb Tenses

To examine (the patient)	Present	Past	Future
Simple	She examines the patient.	She examined the patient.	She will examine the patient.
Progressive	She is examining the patient.	She was examining the patient.	She will be examining the patient.
Perfect	She has examined the patient.	She had examined the patient.	She will have examined the patient.
To draw (the patient's blood)			
Simple	I draw the patient's blood.	I drew the patient's blood.	I will draw the patient's blood.
Progressive	I am drawing the patient's blood.	I was drawing the patient's blood.	I will be drawing the patient's blood.
Perfect	I have drawn the patient's blood.	I had drawn the patient's blood.	I will have drawn the patient's blood.

The progressive tense uses a form of *to be* and the *–ing* form of the verb to show actions that are continuing for a while.

- Ms. Johnson is coming in to the clinic three times this week to receive dialysis.
- Dr. Rodriguez was still examining Mr. Chen when the medical assistant arrived.

| PRACTICE WITH | VERBS AND VERB TENSES |

Underline the correct verb tense in each of the sentences.

1 Mr. Bernard (**came/will come**) in for his pulmonary function test yesterday.

2 As soon as I finish tomorrow's biology test, I (**will go/go**) to my internship site.

3 The patient (**has been waiting/was waiting**) for over an hour now.

4 The last time she was here, Miss Vega (**spoke/has spoken**) to the physical therapist.

5 Dr. Dickenson has not called me yet. I (**am still waiting/still wait**) by the phone.

Section 10-2 (To accompany Chapter 2, "Nonverbal Communication")

Adjectives

Adjectives describe or modify nouns and pronouns. Adjectives can go before nouns or after linking verbs. Adjectives that go after linking verbs are called predicate adjectives. They are called this because the predicate part of a sentence (or clause) includes the verb and objects or phrases connected to the verb. (See the section on Subjects and Predicates later in this chapter.)

- The infected wound needs to be treated. (*Infected* is describing the *wound.*)
- That wound looks infected and needs to be treated. (*Infected* is a predicate adjective that comes after the linking verb *looks* and describes the *wound.*)
- The sleeping patient shouldn't be disturbed. (*Sleeping* is describing the *patient.*)
- The patient is sleeping and shouldn't be disturbed. (*Sleeping* is a predicate adjective that comes after the linking verb *is* and describes the *patient.*)

   Note: Writers should feel comfortable using adjectives in both of these ways. Both methods are equally effective.

Adverbs

Adverbs are words that describe or modify verbs, adjectives, other adverbs, or whole clauses and sentences. They usually end in *–ly.* They often explain the *how, when, where, why,* or *how much* of something that happens in a sentence.

- The phlebotomy nurse washed their hands thoroughly before leaving the patient's room. (The adverb *thoroughly* modifies the verb *washed.*)
- The patient's sprained ankle was very swollen. (The adverb *very* describes the adjective *swollen.*)

- The patient's blood pressure dropped extremely quickly during the surgery. (The adverb *extremely* modifies the adverb *quickly*, which is describing the verb *dropped.*)
- Unfortunately, the patient did not prepare for their positron emission tomography (PET) scan on Monday. (The adverb *unfortunately* modifies the entire sentence.)

PRACTICE WITH ADJECTIVES AND ADVERBS

Identify the words in bold print below as adjectives (ADJ) or adverbs (ADV). Draw an arrow to the word each one modifies or describes.

1 The patient responded **quickly** to the **physical** therapy.
2 During his long convalescence from a **near-fatal** crash, Mr. Simpson made **good** use of his time by learning to speak Spanish **fluently.**
3 The ACE bandage was wrapped **tightly** around Mr. Pilgrim's **left** wrist.
4 The medicine tasted so **bad** that the patient **firmly** refused to take another swallow.
5 The doctor spoke **quietly** with the patient's family about the **upcoming** surgery.

Prepositions and Prepositional Phrases

Prepositions are words that often show relationships of time and space, that is, when or where something takes place.

- The patient interrupted the doctor during the visit. (The preposition *during* tells you *when* the patient interrupted the doctor.)
- The nurse is in the examination room. (The preposition *in* tells you *where* the nurse is.)

Box 10-4 Examples of Prepositions

about	around	by	in front of	on	to
above	before	down	inside	onto	toward
across	behind	during	into	out of	until
after	below	except	like	outside	up
against	beneath	for	near	past	with
along	beside	from	next to	since	within
among	between	in	of	through	without

A *prepositional phrase* is a group of words made up of the preposition and the words that follow it. The noun or pronoun that follows the preposition is called the *object* of the preposition.

- Behind the desk (*Desk* is the object of *behind.*)
- In the hospital (*Hospital* is the object of *in.*)

- With the stethoscope (*Stethoscope* is the object of *with.*)
- Around the wound (*Wound* is the object of *around.*)
- Above the waist (*Waist* is the object of *above.*)
- Through a needle (*Needle* is the object of *through.*)

Prepositional phrases are important parts of sentences. It is usually helpful to remember that the subject of a sentence will not appear in a prepositional phrase.

- The radiology technologist placed the patient's elbow on the table. (*On the table* is a prepositional phrase in this sentence.)
- The nurse looked at the wound during the patient's visit. (This sentence has two prepositional phrases: *at the wound* and *during the patient's visit.*)
- The pharmacist spoke to the patient about the new medication after the doctor's appointment. (This sentence has three prepositional phrases: *to the patient*, *about the new medication*, and *after the doctor's appointment.*)

PRACTICE WITH	PREPOSITIONS AND PREPOSITIONAL PHRASES

Identify the prepositions below by circling them, and then cross out any prepositional phrases.

1 The patient sat in the examination room waiting for the nurse.
2 Martha went to the library to find a book on gingivitis.
3 Both of the medical assistants enjoyed working with the phlebotomy nurse during blood gas draws.
4 After his MRI, Mr. Gilroy hoped to find out what the source of pain was in his right shoulder.
5 Drinking two liters of contrast agent took John 30 minutes. When he was finished, he put the glass down on the bedside table and climbed out of bed.

Conjunctions

Conjunctions are words that join two or more parts of a sentence. They connect words, phrases, or clauses. The two kinds of conjunctions discussed here are coordinating conjunctions and subordinating conjunctions.

Coordinating Conjunctions

Coordinating conjunctions connect two or more words, phrases, or clauses. Coordinating conjunctions include *and, but, for, or, nor, so,* and *yet.*

- The nurse *and* the doctor included notes in the patient's chart. (The coordinating conjunction *and* connects the two words *nurse* and *doctor*.)
- The overworked medical assistant could not decide whether to prepare the examination room or to take the lab samples down to the pathology lab. (The coordinating conjunction *or* links the two phrases *to prepare the examination room* and *to take the lab samples*.)
- All members of the healthcare team went to the conference room for the weekly meeting, but the nurse manager had not arrived yet. (The coordinating conjunction *but* connects the two clauses *all members of the healthcare team went to the conference room for the weekly meeting* and *the nurse manager had not arrived yet*.)
- Mary, the pharmacist, explained the medication's dosage, and she demonstrated how to load the syringe. (The coordinating conjunction *and* connects the two clauses *Mary the pharmacist explained the medication's dosage* and *she demonstrated how to load the syringe*.)

Subordinating Conjunctions

Subordinating conjunctions begin dependent clauses and connect them with independent clauses. (See Dependent and Independent Clauses later in this chapter.) The subordinating conjunction shows the relationship between the two clauses, and generally explains *when, why,* or *under what circumstances*. Below is a list of the most common subordinating conjunctions.

Box 10-5 Examples of Subordinating Conjunctions				
after	as though	if	that	whenever
although	because	once	though	where
as	before	since	unless	whereas
as if	even if	so that	until	wherever
as long as	even though	than	when	while

- When the patient checked in for their appointment, the medical assistant escorted them to the examination room. (*When the patient checked in for their appointment* is a dependent clause. *When* is the subordinating conjunction. *The medical assistant escorted them to the examination room* is an independent clause.)
- Because the patient had not followed the directions to eat a carbohydrate-free/high-protein diet, they were not ready for their PET scan this morning. (*Because the patient had not followed the directions to eat a carbohydrate-free/high-protein diet* is a dependent clause. *Because* is the subordinating conjunction. *They were not ready for their PET scan this morning* is an independent clause.)

PRACTICE WITH CONJUNCTIONS AND PREPOSITIONS

Identify the words in bold print as coordinating conjunctions (CC), subordinating conjunctions (SC), or prepositions (PREP).

1 **When** Mary arrived at the clinic, she turned **on** all the lights **and** unlocked the examination rooms.

2 Mr. Ford came **in** for his physical **after** work.

3 **If** Dr. Rodriguez calls **before** 6 p.m., can you tell him that the patient is **at** the pharmacy waiting **for** the prescription?

4 I don't know the answer **to** that question **about** mitosis, **but** I know all the material **on** meiosis.

5 Can you explain the difference **between** white blood cells **and** red blood cells?

6 Mary has worked **as** a nurse **in** this clinic **since** she passed her licensure examination **in** 1997.

7 **Because** he was careful not to violate any of the hospital's patient privacy policies, Andrew told the newspaper reporters he could not confirm or deny **that** the star quarterback was currently undergoing knee surgery. He directed all calls **to** the hospital's public relations office **on** the fifth floor.

8 **During** the long surgery, the patient's family waited **in** the reception area eating cookies **and** drinking coffee.

9 **After** he finished answering the test's multiple choice questions, Barry began answering the short answer **and** matching questions.

10 David held the stethoscope **against** the mannequin's chest, **but** he could not hear a heartbeat.

Section 10-3 (To accompany Chapter 3, "Verbal Communication")

Punctuation

Punctuation helps you to be clear in your writing. Punctuation marks show relationships within a sentence and show the reader where the sentence ends.

Periods

Use periods at the ends of sentences, in abbreviations, and in decimals. These are examples of periods ending sentences.

■ The doctor examined the patient.

■ The medical assistant took the patient's vital signs.
■ Sneezing is one symptom of allergies.

These are examples of periods used in abbreviations.

Box 10-6 Examples of Periods in Abbreviations

Dr.	Mr.	Ms.	Mrs.	M.D.	R.N.	L.P.N.	N.A.	M.A.	M.S.
B.S.	B.A.	a.m.	p.m.	J.D.	Inc.	Co.	Corp.	Blvd.	Ave.

Remember that medical abbreviations can appear in upper or lower case letters and with or without a period. When you write measurements, be sure *not* to use periods.

Box 10-7 Medical Abbreviations and Measurements

b.i.d.	a.c.	h.s.	MI	PFT	CBC	Hb	WBC	ETOH	
mm	cm	ml	l	cl	mcg	mg	kg	oz	ft

Use periods in decimals and to separate dollars and cents.

■ My GPA is 3.49.
■ He measured 0.56 cm.
■ The per-visit co-pay is $10.50.

Question Marks and Exclamation Marks

Like periods, question marks and exclamation marks are used to end sentences. Each, however, is used to end a different kind of sentence.

Question Marks

Use a question mark at the end of a direct question.

■ Do you feel any pain when I press your abdomen here?
■ When did you first notice the ringing in your ears?
■ Will the nurse draw any blood this evening?
■ Does Mr. Jones have a living will?

Exclamation Marks

Use an exclamation mark to end a sentence showing urgency, emotion, or excitement.

■ Call a code blue in Room C223!
■ Take these bloods to the lab STAT!
■ Do not let anyone except the doctor into that room!
■ He survived a quadruple bypass!

| PRACTICE WITH | PERIODS, QUESTION MARKS, AND EXCLAMATION MARKS |

Proofread and correct the following passage, adding periods, question marks, and exclamation marks where necessary. You should find eight (8) errors to correct.

David, a medical assistant, was working on Saturday at the nursing station in the Department of Hematology/Oncology Part of his job was to greet patients' friends and family members who came to the department on visits.

At about 10 a.m., an elderly woman came up to the nursing station with a question She was a short woman who had to stand on her toes to see over the desk to speak to David. She seemed very confused.

Do you know where the Department of Cardiology is" she asked. "Is this the Department of Cardiology."

David knew that Cardiology was over in the next wing of the hospital and two floors up. He worried that if he gave the woman directions, she might get lost again He wanted to provide the best service possible to her.

It's quite a ways from here," he said. "I'd be happy to escort you there to make sure you find it."

The elderly woman smiled a bright smile to David "Thank you so much That's the nicest thing anyone's done for me today"

Commas

The comma, one of the most frequently used and misused pieces of punctuation, makes clear the relationships within a sentence.

Lists
Use commas between items in a list.

- The medical assistant noticed that the office first-aid kit lacked bandages, tape, gauze, and alcohol pads.
- The nursing student brought books, notepads, pens, and rulers.

Note: In academic writing, be sure to use the final comma before the conjunction in a list (*and, but, yet, nor, or*).

Coordinate Adjectives
Use a comma between two adjectives that could be separated by *and*. Note that coordinate adjectives all modify the *same* noun.

- The basketball player came into the coach's office with a red, swollen knee. (The same sentence could be written with *and* between *red* and *swollen*.)
- James's asthma has shown a slow, steady improvement. (The same sentence could be written with *and* between *slow* and *steady*.)

Introductory Phrases or Clauses

Use a comma after an introductory phrase or a dependent clause.

- To help chemotherapy patients understand possible dietary restrictions, the American Cancer Society has produced this excellent pamphlet.
- Because the American Cancer Society has produced this excellent pamphlet, chemotherapy patients can have a better understanding of possible dietary restrictions.

Note: If the independent clause comes before the dependent clause, do not use a comma.

- Chemotherapy patients can have a better understanding of possible dietary restrictions because the American Cancer Society produced this excellent pamphlet.

Coordinating Conjunctions

Use a comma before a coordinating conjunction (*and, but, or, for, nor, so, yet*) in a sentence with two independent clauses, called a *compound sentence.* (See Independent Clauses later in this chapter)

- James's asthma is much improved, *but* it is still not completely controlled. (This sentence has two independent clauses: *James's asthma is much improved* and *it is still not completely controlled.*)
- James's asthma is not completely controlled, *yet* it is much improved. (This sentence has two independent clauses: *James's asthma is not completely controlled* and *it is much improved.*)
- James's asthma is much improved, *and* he will continue to see Dr. Rodriguez for more treatment. (This sentence has two independent clauses: *James's asthma is much improved* and *he will continue to see Dr. Rodriguez for more treatment.*)

Nonessential Clauses

Use commas around nonessential dependent clauses. Do not put commas around essential clauses. A clause is nonessential if you can take it out of the sentence without changing the sentence's meaning. The commas around the nonessential clause tell the reader that this clause contains extra, nonessential information.

- James, who is an avid video game player, is taking a new cortisone inhaler to control his asthma. (The clause *who is an avid video game player* is nonessential to the meaning of the sentence.)
- That cabinet, which the maintenance staff installed last week, contains all of the surgical prep kits we have left. (The clause *which the maintenance staff installed last week* is nonessential to the meaning of the sentence.)

You should not put commas around a clause that is essential to a sentence. The lack of commas tells the reader that the information in the clause is essential to the basic meaning of the sentence.

- The doctor who ordered this medication for James is not in the hospital today. (The clause *who ordered this medication for James* is essential to the meaning of the sentence. Without this information, the reader would not know which doctor the writer is referring to.)
- The medical records that contained the x-ray report were on the table in the conference room. (The clause *that contained the x-ray report* is essential to meaning of the sentence. Without this information, the reader would not know which medical records the writer is referring to.)

Note: Use the following guideline when deciding whether to use *which* or *that* to introduce a clause. Use *which* for a **nonessential** clause, and use *that* for an **essential** clause. Remember always to use *who* when referring to a person.

- The department of cardiology, **which is on the East end of the fourth floor,** is staffed by a team of dedicated healthcare professionals. (The clause *which is on the East end of the fourth floor* is nonessential to the meaning of the sentence. Note that the clause is set off by commas.)
- The only department **that has an open bed for the incoming patient** is cardiology. (The clause *that has an open bed for the incoming patient* is essential to the meaning of the sentence. Without this information, the sentence would read *The only department is cardiology,* and the reader would not understand what the writer means.)

Appositive Phrases
Use commas around appositive phrases. (These are phrases that modify or describe nouns or pronouns with different words.)

- Jennifer Martinez, the nursing assistant who is on duty this evening, will check to see that all examination rooms are stocked with alcohol prep pads. (The phrase *the nursing assistant who is on duty this evening* identifies Jennifer Martinez by describing her.)
- Mr. Nguyen, a geriatric patient of Dr. Jones's, is coming in with his daughter today. (The phrase *a geriatric patient of Dr. Jones's* identifies Mr. Nguyen by describing him.)

Clarity
Use commas to make the meaning of your sentences clearer.

- **Unclear:** To Dr. Scott James was a pleasant patient because of his compliant and easy-going behavior.

- **Clear:** To Dr. Scott, James was a pleasant patient because of his compliant and easy-going behavior.

Other Uses for Commas
Also use commas in the following situations:

In addresses and geographic place names

- The clinic is at 1655 Highland Avenue, Glendale, California.
- Dr. Rodriguez did his residency in Glendale, Arizona, not Glendale, California.

In openings and closings of letters and emails

- Dear Ms. Johnson,
- Sincerely,

When you directly address another person

- Dr. Rodriguez, do you have the patient's medical record with you?
- Marcel, do you know where Dr. Rodriguez did his residency?

To separate a name from a title or degree and with Jr. and Sr.

- Be sure to address the letter to Michael Chen, M.D.
- Be sure to label the chart Carlos Ramirez, Jr. Carlos Ramirez, Sr. is his father.

In dates

- His date of birth is March 24, 1988.
- I was hired on International Nurses Day, which was May 12, 2010.

With numbers that have more than three digits.

- She donated $5,000 to the hospital charity.
- The plane delivered 2,000,000 flu shot ampules last week.

PRACTICE WITH COMMAS

Proofread the following passage. Add commas where necessary. You should add at least 23 commas.

Michael a first-year nursing student has a medical terminology exam and a biology paper due tomorrow. He has been studying medical terminology all week and he has written much of the paper. In fact the biology paper is almost finished. Michael figures that he has four maybe five more hours to work on it. He has just arrived in the library with his book bag. In the book bag he has his laptop computer his biology textbook his medical terminology textbook his note cards and his notebooks. If he finishes his biology paper he will not have enough time to study for his medical terminology exam. If he studies for medical terminology he will not have enough time to write his biology paper.

The library is crowded. After 15 minutes of looking around the library Michael cannot find an open seat at any of the tables or cubicles. The school has just over 7000 students and it seems to Michael that at least 6999 of them are already there in the library.

After another 10 minutes of looking Michael decides to go back to his room. His room is cramped cluttered and crowded. Still he figures that if he stays up all night he might have enough time to finish the biology paper and study for his medical terminology exam. It's going to be a long long night.

Section 10-4 (To accompany Chapter 4, "Professional Communication and Behavior")

Semicolons

Use semicolons to connect parts of a sentence in the following ways.

Independent Clauses without Conjunctions

Use a semicolon to connect two independent clauses that are not connected by a coordinating conjunction (*and*, *but*, *for*, *or*, *nor*, *so*, and *yet*) but are closely related.

- Ms. Augustin is calling for her test results; she had her bloods drawn last week. (The two ideas are closely related.)
- Dr. Clarke said she needed these blood cultures taken to the lab STAT; the patient is running a high fever. (The two ideas are closely related.)

Independent Clauses with Conjunctive Adverbs

Use a semicolon to connect independent clauses that are joined by a conjunctive adverb (*however*, *nevertheless*, *moreover*, *therefore*) or transitional phrases (*as a result*, *for example*).

- James's asthma is much improved; however, he still has trouble breathing in cold weather.
- The nursing supervisor has come up with many great ideas for improving patient care; for example, she suggested that the triage nurse speak to patients by phone before they arrive.

Items in a Long List

Use semicolons in a long list of items, especially if there are commas within some of the items.

- Please be sure that the first aid kit includes bandages, both adhesive and non-adhesive; tape; gauze; non-latex gloves; alcohol wipes; and cotton swabs, especially that kind with wooden sticks.

Colons

Use a colon to present specific, important information.

Before a List, a Series, or a Quotation

■ On the day of the exam, each nursing student should bring the following: one black pen, two blue books, a ruler, a stethoscope, and the exam study guide.

■ Dr. Joe Shamir captured the spirit of our clinic's mission when he said on this day in 1976: "All of our patients deserve the very best care we can provide. That must be our number one priority. Nothing matters more than providing patients with the best care humanly and economically possible."

Other Uses for Colons
After the salutation in a formal letter or memorandum

■ Dear Dr. Rodriguez:
■ Dear Ms. Jones:
■ To: Nursing Staff, 2CW

In the writing of time

■ The doctor will arrive at 3:15 promptly.
■ I've been waiting for the patient since 8:00.

| PRACTICE WITH | SEMICOLONS AND COLONS |

Proofread the following passage from a letter, adding semicolons and colons where necessary. You should find at least eight (8) places to correct errors.

Dear Mr. Pierre

At 915 last Wednesday morning, I called your office to ask about the status of my application for the open nursing assistant position that was advertised in *the Herald*. I left a message with Jane, the receptionist, who told me she would return my call later that day however, a week has passed, and I have not heard back yet. I believe my credentials closely match those listed in the advertisement an associate's degree in a health-related major 2 years experience working in a healthcare setting a desire to help patients, especially elderly patients and basic telephone and computer skills.

I would very much like to discuss with you the ways I may contribute to Longmeadow Medical Associates. I can be reached at my home phone 818-987-9876.

Sincerely,
Melanie Johnston

Apostrophes

Use apostrophes to show possessives and contractions.

Possessives

Use an apostrophe to show that a noun or indefinite pronoun is possessive.

Singular Nouns
Use -*'s* with singular nouns and pronouns.

- *Mrs. Nguyen's* medical record has been completely updated.
- *Everyone's* computer password will be reset next week.

Plural Nouns
Use –*s'* with plural nouns that form the plural by adding an *s*.

- All of the patients' records have been completely updated.
- Can you tell me where the nurses' report room is?

Two or More Nouns
Use -*'s* on the last noun to show joint ownership, and on each noun to show individual ownership.

- Susan and Barbara's car is parked behind the clinic. (Joint ownership)
- John's and Barbara's lab coats are still at the dry cleaners. (Individual ownership)

Important Note: Possessive pronouns already show possession, so they never take apostrophes.

Box 10-8 Possessive Pronouns						
Followed by a noun:	my	his	her	its	your	their
Not followed by a noun:	mine	his	hers	its	yours	theirs

- This is my book. (The possessive pronoun *my* is followed by a noun, *book*.)
- This book is mine. (The possessive pronoun *mine* is not followed by a noun.)
- The patient's diet is their responsibility. (The possessive pronoun *their* is followed by a noun, *responsibility*.)
- The responsibility for the patient's diet is theirs (The possessive pronoun *theirs* is not followed by a noun.

Hyphens

Hyphens are important for clarity, and should be used in the following ways.

Compound Modifiers
Use a hyphen to punctuate compound words that work together as adjectives to modify a noun.

- Mr. Wright needs to be scheduled for a *follow-up* appointment.
- I looked closely at the *grayish-black* area around the wound.
- The patient's father gave the doctor *second-hand* information.

Do not use a hyphen if the compound modifier follows the noun.

- I looked closely at the surrounding tissue, which was grayish black.
- The doctor heard the information second hand.

Note: When the first word in a compound modifier is an adverb (ending in *–ly*) or *very*, do not use a hyphen.

- Dr. Martin is an *internationally* known cardiologist.
- I looked closely at the *partially* removed tissue.
- Jennifer is a *very* sweet nurse.

Compound Words

Use a hyphen to form a compound word. A compound word has more than one word in it but works as a single word.

- John's *sister-in-law* is studying for her licensure examination.
- Dr. Rodriguez may seem like a *happy-go-lucky* guy, but he is really a very serious person.

Prefixes

Use a hyphen to connect many prefixes to words. Common hyphenated prefixes include *ex-*, *pro-*, *self-*.

- The ex-president of the American Medical Association is going to speak at the seminar.
- The Surgeon General did not make a distinction between those who were pro-life and those who were pro-choice.

Note: Always be sure to use a dictionary to see if you should use a hyphen with a prefix.

Other Uses for a Hyphen

- In written fractions: *one-fifth, two-thirds, one-fifteenth*
- In numbers from *twenty-one* to *ninety-nine*
- In numbers and dates that indicate a span of time: *1990-1998, 6:00-7:30*

PRACTICE WITH APOSTROPHES AND HYPHENS

Proofread the following sentences. Insert apostrophes and hyphens where needed.

1 Mrs. Smiths daughter in law is coming in to meet with Dr. Rodriguez to discuss Mrs. Smiths care plan.

2 Dr. Chen always sees the glass as half full. Dr. Johnson sees the glass as half empty. However, Dr. Chens nurse sees the glass as two thirds full.

3 Meghan came to visit Cara 23 times last week after Caras appendix was removed.

4 Dr. Martin wants to have a face to face meeting with Mr. Hernandez's future son in law.

5 One half of all babies born from 1960 1970 were inoculated.

Dashes

In some cases, you can use dashes instead of commas.

- For Parenthetical Information: *Mrs. Pontiac – the patient whose family always brings in a huge batch of chocolate chip cookies big enough for the entire nursing staff – has followed her sugar-free diet carefully.*
- For Lists and Explanations: *Mr. Lee asked for a complete list of what we do when we check vitals – blood pressure, respiratory rate, body temperature, and pulse rate.*

Parentheses

You can use parentheses in a few important ways.

- Around extra, additional information: *Mrs. Pontiac (the best baker in town) is on a strict sugar-free diet.*
- Around information that explains: *Mrs. Pontiac's third son (the one who started a bake shop on Fifth Avenue) has a monopoly on the market for chocolate chip cookies in Savannah.*
- Around numbers or letters in lists within sentences: *Remember to check Mr. Santiago's vitals: (1) pulse rate, (2) respiratory rate, (3) blood pressure, and (4) body temperature.*

Quotation Marks

Use quotation marks to enclose the exact words of a speaker or writer. You may need to use quotation marks to quote the exact words of a patient or family member.

- "Mark's behavior has become increasingly erratic over the past months," Mr. Smith said about his son.
- The patient said to his nurse, "I have a dull, heavy pain in my chest and a tingling in my neck and chin."
- "Never do harm" is part of the Hippocratic Oath.

Also use quotation marks to show part of a published work, such as a chapter, or to indicate that words or phrases are used in a particular way.

- The last chapter in this book is called "Fundamental Writing Skills."
- Write "Return to Sender" on the envelope.
- Put a sign on the door that says "Meeting in Progress."

Capital Letters

Use capital letters at the start of sentences, in proper nouns, in titles, and for adjectives derived from proper nouns.

Proper Nouns
Use capital letters to begin names of people, races, titles, geographical locations, months, seasons, and organizations. Do not use capital letters for general names of these things.

- The Mayo Clinic (a specific name) is the best clinic (a general name) in the state.
- President Simpson (a specific name) is the seventh president (a general name) this HMO has had in the last 5 years.
- Massachusetts has many great hospitals (a general name); the Brigham and Women's Hospital (a specific name) is just one of the best known.

Titles
Use capital letters to begin all words in titles except for articles (*the, a, an*), prepositions (e.g., *in, through, across, after*), and conjunctions (e.g., *and* or *but*). If an article, preposition, or conjunction is the first word of the title, you should capitalize it.

- *The Heirs of General Practice* is my favorite book by John McPhee.
- "The Use of Force" is one of *The Doctor Stories* by William Carlos Williams.

Other Uses for Capital Letters
Always use capital letters when writing the following:

- Nations and Countries: United States of America, Mexico, Kenya, Haiti, Ukraine
- Planets: Earth, Mars, Jupiter
- Public place names: Copley Square, Ellis Island, Zuma Beach
- Names of streets: Broadway, Highland Avenue, Primrose Lane
- Days of week and names of months: Thursday, Sunday, March, September
- Holidays: Thanksgiving, Memorial Day, Martin Luther King, Jr. Day

- Religions: Catholicism, Buddhism, Judaism, Islam
- Languages: English, Spanish, German, Mandarin, Creole
- The first-person pronoun (always): I

Note: Always check a dictionary if you do not know whether a word or phrase should have capital letters.

PRACTICE WITH | **QUOTATION MARKS AND CAPITAL LETTERS**

Proofread the following sentences. Add quotation marks and capital letters where appropriate.

1 Suzanne has just published an article entitled meeting new patients' needs in the latest issue of *the journal of nursing*.
2 Mr. Keller's exact words were: just try to give me that flu shot. i'll show you.
3 Cheryl is going to madrid, spain, for thanksgiving.
4 The former president wanted to do more to restructure the hmo than president Cranston does.
5 Before he went in for his abdominal surgery, Mr. Martinez kept singing that old beatles song Don't let me down.

Numbers

Ordinal Numbers and Cardinal Numbers

Box 10-9 Ordinal Numbers and Cardinal Numbers

Ordinal numbers show the order in which something happens.

Ordinal Numbers

Examples of ordinal numbers written as numerals are
1st, 2nd, 3rd, 5th, 10th, 15th, 21st, 22nd, 30th, 41st, 43rd, 52nd, 61st, 74th, 76th, 87th, 93rd, 99th, 100th

Examples of ordinal numbers written as words are
first, second, third, fifth, twenty-first, twenty-eighth, thirtieth, forty-third, fifty-fourth, sixty-seventh, seventy-sixth, ninety-ninth, one-hundredth

Cardinal Numbers

Examples of cardinal numbers written as numerals are
1, 2, 3, 5, 10, 15, 21, 22, 30, 41, 43, 52, 61, 74, 76, 87, 93, 99, 100

Examples of cardinal numbers written as words are
one, two, three, five, ten, twenty-one, twenty-two, thirty, forty-three, fifty-two, sixty-one, seventy-six, ninety-nine, one hundred

Arabic Numerals and Roman Numerals

Box 10-10 Arabic Numerals and Roman Numerals

Arabic Numerals	Roman Numerals	Arabic Numerals	Roman Numerals
1	I	20	XX
2	II	30	XXX
3	III	40	XL
4	IV	50	L
5	V	60	LX
6	VI	70	LXX
7	VII	80	LXXX
8	VIII	90	XC
9	IX	100	C
10	X	200	CC
11	XI	300	CCC
12	XII	400	CD
13	XIII	500	D
14	XIV	600	DC
15	XV	700	DCC
16	XVI	800	DCCC
17	XVII	900	CM
18	XVIII	1,000	M
19	XIX		

Use the following guidelines when writing numbers as words or as numerals.

Box 10-11 Guidelines for Writing Numbers as *Words* or as *Numerals*

Write numbers as words in these situations:

- When the number is ten or lower: one, two, four, seven, nine, ten.
- When the number is the first word in a sentence: Twenty-one blood cultures were run.
- When the number is an indefinite number: a couple hundred, a few million.
- When the number is a fraction alone in a sentence: He gave me one-third of the pie.
- When the date is an ordinal number with no month: Tomorrow is my twenty-first birthday.
- When you use words for numbers everywhere else in the phrase, clause or sentence: The doctor ordered two blood cultures and three urine samples in the next twenty-four hours.
- When you use a number under 10 in a name: She lives on Fifth Avenue.

Write numbers as numerals in these situations:

- When the number is over ten: 11, 15, 22, 27, 99.
- When you indicate a patient's age: The patient is 48 years old.
- When you use numerals everywhere else in the phrase, clause or sentence: The patient in the emergency room received 157 stitches, 22 staples, and 3 small bandages on their back.

(continued)

Box 10-11 Guidelines for Writing Numbers as *Words* or as *Numerals* (continued)

- When you use separate, unrelated numbers with a comma: On March 22, 112 people visited the emergency room.
- When you use numbers with symbols and abbreviations: 55%, #16 gauge needle, 10 cc, pH 7.5, 100 mg.
- When you write drug amounts: 1 mg of Alprazolam, 50 mcg of Fluticasone Propionate.
- When the day precedes the month, write the date as an ordinal: the 5th of May.
- When you indicate amounts of money: $25, $9.95, 50 cents (Note: Always use the word cents for amounts under a dollar. Use the dollar sign for amounts over a dollar. Do not include .00 with even dollar amounts.)
- When you indicate a time with a.m. or p.m.: 10:15 a.m., 7:30 p.m. (Note: Do not use :00 with exact hour times 6 a.m., 9 p.m. Do not use a.m. or p.m. with the word o'clock: 8 o'clock.)
- When you indicate numbers that have decimal fractions: 6.5 cm, 1.5 l. (Note: Always include a zero before a decimal that is not a whole number: 0.4 mg, 0.6%.
- When you indicate dimensions, sizes, and temperatures as numerals: He wears a 10½ size shoe. It's 10 degrees below zero.

PRACTICE WITH NUMBERS

Proofread the following sentences. Make any corrections necessary with numbers.

1 78 patients were sitting in the lobby for thirty minutes waiting for flu shots.
2 Marcia is very good at drawing blood. I'm sure she's drawn blood from a few 100 patients this year.
3 The article said that fifty-five % of newborns in that state had fewer than 2 siblings.
4 The new suture kits cost thirty-nine dollars each.
5 Dr. Rashad said he would be here at ten a.m. sharp.

Section 10-5 (To accompany Chapter 5, "Interviewing Techniques")

Sentence Grammar

Effective communicators in any profession need to understand the parts of sentences and how they work together.

Subjects and Predicates

Subjects and predicates are the two parts of a sentence. The *simple* subject is the who or what the sentence is about, and the *simple* predicate shows the action (or, with linking verbs, what is called *the state of being.*)

■ The EMT arrived. (*EMT* is the subject; *arrived* is the predicate.)
■ The patient is eating. (*Patient* is the subject; *is eating* is the predicate.)

A sentence can become more complicated when it includes other words, phrases, and clauses that modify the subject and the predicate, forming what is called a *complete* subject and *complete* predicate.

■ The phlebotomy nurse went into Room 215C to take a blood gas on Mr. Jimenez. (*The phlebotomy nurse* is the **complete subject,** and the **complete predicate** is *went into Room 215C to take a blood gas on Mr. Jimenez.*)
■ The patient in the examination room wants to talk to Dr. Chen before leaving. (*The patient in the examination room* is the **complete subject,** and the **complete predicate** is *wants to talk to Dr. Chen before leaving.*)
■ The plastic syringes in that box don't have proper labeling. (*The plastic syringes in that box* is the **complete subject,** and the **complete predicate** is *don't have proper labeling.*)

PRACTICE WITH   SUBJECTS AND PREDICATES

Identify the complete subjects (CS) and complete predicates (CP) in each sentence.

1 The patient survived.
2 These medications control James's asthma.
3 Mr. Adjani will call Dr. Williamson tomorrow morning about the test results.
4 The examination rooms are all clean.
5 Dr. Rodriguez is the only cardiologist who came out for the hospital charity's Valentine's Day party.

Phrases

A phrase is a group of words without a subject or a verb. A phrase never expresses a complete thought but always modifies a noun or a verb. Phrases are important parts of most sentences.

Prepositional Phrases
Prepositional phrases are the most common kind of phrases in English. A prepositional phrase contains a preposition and its object (the noun or pronoun in the phrase).

- The nurse looked at the patient's hands. (*At the patient's hands* is the prepositional phrase.)
- Dr. Schmidt will look at the patient's chart before he goes into the examination room. (*At the patient's chart* and *into the examination room* are prepositional phrases.)
- *Across the River and into the Trees* is one of my favorite books by Hemingway. (*Across the River* and *into the Trees* are both prepositional phrases.)

Verbal Phrases

Verbal phrases are formed by verbs but work as nouns or modifiers. The three types of verbal phrases include *infinitives*, *gerunds*, and *participles*.

Infinitive Phrases

Infinitives are formed by adding *to* in front of the verb (to examine, to write, to communicate). An infinitive phrase contains the infinitive and its modifiers.

- Jessica went to the library to study her nursing homework. (*To study her nursing homework* is the infinitive phrase.)
- Mrs. Ngogi came to the clinic to have her blood pressure taken. (*To have her blood pressure taken* is the infinitive phrase.)

Gerund Phrases

A gerund is formed by adding *–ing* to a verb. Gerunds work as nouns in sentences, frequently as the subject or direct object. A gerund phrase includes its modifiers.

- Understanding the principles of effective communication is important if you want to succeed professionally. (*Understanding the principles of effective communication* is a gerund phrase that works as the subject of the sentence.)
- Eating plenty of fruits and vegetables is a part of any healthy diet. (*Eating plenty of fruits and vegetables* is a gerund phrase working as the subject of the sentence.)
- Dr. Fritz likes examining patients who speak German. (*Examining patients* is a gerund phrase that works as a direct object of the verb *like*s.)

Participles

Participles are formed by adding *–ing* in present tense or *–ed* in past tense to verbs. They work as adjectives that modify nouns or pronouns. A participle phrase includes its modifiers.

- The patient, sitting on the examination table, told the nurse her medical history. (*Sitting on the examination table* is a present participle modifying the subject of the sentence, the noun *patient.*)

■ Covering her eyes with her hands, she walked out of the conference room where her colleagues had gathered for a surprise birthday party (*Covering her eyes with her hands* is a present participle modifying the subject of the sentence, the pronoun *she.*).
■ Exhausted from studying all night for her biology exam, Barbara wanted to stop for another cup of coffee on her way to class. (*Exhausted from studying all night for her biology exam* is a past participle modifying the subject of the sentence, the noun *Barbara.*)

PRACTICE WITH PHRASES

In the sentences below, identify the phrases in bold print as prepositional (P), infinitive (I), gerund (G), or participial (Part).

1 Mr. Vieira did not say a word to me **during the entire physical examination.**
2 **Skipping meals** is not a healthy way **to lose weight.**
3 Fists clenched, the little boy screamed **at the nurse** who had given him a shot **in his arm.**
4 **Helping patients better understand their treatment options** is the only responsible course to take.
5 Mrs. O'Donnell's daughter-in-law went out to the lobby to wait **during the 3-hour procedure.**

Clauses

A clause is a group of words that contains both a subject and a verb. Clauses can be independent clauses or dependent (also called subordinate) clauses.

Independent Clauses

An independent clause expresses a complete idea. An independent clause can stand alone as a complete sentence or as part of a longer sentence.

■ Three staff members were late today. (This is an independent clause – a complete sentence.)
■ Three staff members were late today because of a breakdown on the subway line. (*Three members were late today* is an independent clause in a longer sentence.)
■ The patient seemed confused. (This is an independent clause – a complete sentence.)
■ When the doctor asked her about taking her medication, the patient seemed confused. (*The patient seemed confused* is an independent clause in a longer sentence.)

Dependent Clauses

A dependent clause (also called a subordinate clause) cannot stand alone as a complete sentence. A dependent clause always has a subject and a verb, but it does not express a complete thought. A dependent clause has to be connected to an independent clause for its full meaning to be clear. A dependent clause always begins with a subordinating conjunction (*if, when, because, while,* and *although* are some examples) or a relative pronoun (*who, whom, that* or *which*).

- Three staff members were late today because of a breakdown on the subway line. (*Because of a breakdown on the subway line* is a dependent clause that needs the independent clause *three staff members were late today* to form a complete sentence.)
- When the doctor asked her about taking her medication, Mrs. Jones seemed confused. (*When the doctor asked her about taking her medication* is a dependent clause that needs the independent clause *Mrs. Jones seemed confused* to form a complete sentence.)
- Josephine Martinique, who studied physical therapy with Dr. Johnson in Boston, is the strongest candidate for the new job opening. (*Who studied physical therapy with Dr. Johnson in Boston* is a dependent clause that needs the independent clause *Josephine Martinique is the strongest candidate for the new job opening* to form a complete sentence.)

PRACTICE WITH **INDEPENDENT AND DEPENDENT CLAUSES**

Identify the clauses in bold print as either independent (I) or dependent (D).

1 **If Mrs. Robertson can come for her physical on Thursday morning at 11:00,** Dr. Rodriguez has an opening on his schedule.
2 **Mr. Solomon needs to go down to radiology for his chest CT.**
3 **The patient's prescription won't be ready for an hour** because the whole computer system went down and a backlog has formed.
4 Patients won't know about the women's health workshop **unless we tell them.**
5 **I don't know** where Dr. Marin put her stethoscope.

Section 10-6 (To accompany Chapter 6, "Adapting Communication to the Patient's Ability to Understand")

Sentence Types

Use phrases and clauses to build clear and effective sentences. The three main kinds of sentences are simple, compound, and complex. All sentences use one of these three types.

Simple Sentences

A simple sentence has one independent clause. A simple sentence can be as short as two words, using just a subject and a verb. A simple sentence can also be longer, using many modifiers and phrases but never any other clauses.

■ Alex studied. (This is a simple sentence – an independent clause – with a subject and a verb.)

■ On Monday afternoon Dr. Fredrickson consulted with radiology on Mrs. Lee's CT scan. (This is a simple sentence with three prepositional phrases: *Dr. Fredrickson* and *consulted* are the subject and verb, and *on Monday afternoon*, *with radiology* and *on Mrs. Lee's CT scan* are all prepositional phrases.)

Compound Sentences

A compound sentence has at least two independent clauses connected by a comma and then a coordinating conjunction (*and, but, for, or, nor, so,* or *yet*).

■ Jermaine was downstairs at the pathology lab waiting, but the patient's unit of type O red blood wasn't ready. (*Jermaine was downstairs at the pathology lab waiting* and *the patient's unit of type O red blood wasn't ready* are both independent clauses, connected by a *comma* and then the coordinating conjunction *but.*)

■ John read the doctor's orders, and then he called the pharmacy to make sure the patient's prescriptions were filled. (*John read the doctor's orders* and *then he called the pharmacy to make sure the patient's prescriptions were filled* are both independent clauses, connected by a *comma* and then the coordinating conjunction *and.*)

A compound sentence can also have three independent clauses.

■ Mr. Ortiz came in for his appointment, and then he began asking frantically for a drink of water, but he said he wasn't thirsty. (*Mr. Ortiz came in for his appointment* and *then he began asking frantically for a drink of water* and *he said he wasn't thirsty* are all independent clauses, connected by *commas* and the coordinating conjunctions *and* and *but.*)

Complex Sentences

A complex sentence has one independent clause and at least dependent clause. The dependent clause will always begin with a subordinating conjunction (*when, if, because, although*) or a relative pronoun (*who, which, that*).

■ We will take Mr. Santos off the neutropenic diet when his white blood cell count rises to an acceptable level. (*We will take Mr. Santos off the neutropenic diet* is an independent clause, and *when his white blood cell count rises to an acceptable level* is a dependent clause started with the subordinating conjunction *when.*)

- Although Mrs. Kenney showed up on time for her colonoscopy, she hadn't prepared by fasting since the evening before. (*Although Mrs. Kenney showed up on time for her colonoscopy* is a dependent clause started with the subordinating conjunction *although,* and *she hadn't prepared by fasting since the evening before* is an independent clause.)

Sentence Errors

You should recognize early on what kinds of errors you might make when writing sentences. Learning how to identify these errors and correct them can help you become a much more effective writer. Here are a few important grammar points to remember, along with some of the most common sentence errors.

Subject-Verb Agreement Errors

A subject and a verb in a sentence must agree in number. If a subject is singular, the verb must be singular. If a subject is plural, the verb must be plural.

When a subject and verb in a sentence do not agree in number, the sentence contains a subject-verb agreement (S-V agreement) error.

- **With S-V Agreement Error:** Mr. Garbo have not completed his medical history forms. — The subject and verb do not agree: the subject *Mr. Garbo* is singular; the verb *have* is plural.
- **Correct Version:** Mr. Garbo has not completed his medical history forms. — The subject and verb agree.
- **With S-V Agreement Error:** The faculty member do a good job helping students learn correct grammar. — The subject and verb do not agree: the subject *faculty member* is singular; the verb *do* is plural.
- **Correct Version:** The faculty member does a good job helping students learn correct grammar. — The subject and verb agree.
- **With S-V Agreement Error:** Studying every day for many hours have made Mark a good medical assisting student but a boring friend. — The subject and verb do not agree: the gerund phrase *studying for many hours* is the subject and is singular; the verb *have* is plural.
- **Correct Version:** Studying every day for many hours has made Mark a good medical assisting student but a boring friend. — The subject and verb agree.

The following indefinite pronouns often serve as subjects in sentences, and all of them are singular: *each, everyone, everybody, everything, either, neither, anyone, anything, anybody, nobody,* and *nothing.*

- **With S-V Agreement Error:** Neither of the doctors are on the cardiology unit. — The subject and verb do not agree: the subject *neither* is singular and the verb *are* is plural.
- **Correct Version:** Neither of the doctors is on the cardiology unit. — The subject and verb agree.

Tip: Remember from the section on prepositions earlier in the chapter that the subject of a sentence will never be in a prepositional phrase — *of the doctors* and *on the cardiology unit* are both prepositional phrases.

PRACTICE WITH SUBJECT-VERB AGREEMENT

In the sentences below, choose the correct verb.

1 Both of the patients (**is/are**) in the examination rooms.
2 Bringing in family members to speak with the healthcare team members (**is/are**) what many elderly patients do to help them understand their treatment options.
3 Neither of the nurses (**has/have**) seen the patients' test results.
4 Many of the patients in this practice (**prefers/prefer**) the early morning schedule.
5 Each of the physicians in the department (**sees/see**) over 50 patients per week.

Run-ons — Fused Sentences and Comma Splice Errors

A run-on occurs when two or more complete sentences are run together without adequate punctuation between them. There are two kinds of run-ons: *fused sentences* and *comma splice errors.*

A fused sentence has no punctuation between two complete sentences.

Fused Sentence: David spent 30 minutes with Mrs. Briggs in her hospital room he came out and wrote three pages of notes on the encounter. (*Dave spent 30 minutes with Mrs. Briggs in her hospital room* and *He came out and wrote three pages of notes on the encounter* are both complete sentences.)

A comma splice error has a comma between two complete sentences. A comma is not adequate punctuation between two complete sentences without a conjunction.

Comma Splice Error: David spent 30 minutes with Mrs. Briggs in her hospital room, he came out and wrote three pages of notes on the encounter.

To correct the error, you must first identify the two complete sentences. Then you can choose one of four ways to complete the correct version.

1 Add a period between the two complete sentences and capitalize the first letter of the second sentence.

David spent 30 minutes with Mrs. Briggs in her hospital room. He came out and wrote three pages of notes on the encounter.

2 Add a semicolon between the two complete sentences. (When you use a semicolon, you do not need to capitalize the first letter in the second sentence.)

David spent 30 minutes with Mrs. Briggs in her hospital room; he came out and wrote three pages of notes on the encounter.

3 Add a comma and a coordinating conjunction between the two complete sentences.

David spent 30 minutes with Mrs. Briggs in her hospital room, and he came out and wrote three pages of notes on the encounter.

4 Add a subordinating conjunction to one of the complete sentences.

After David spent 30 minutes with Mrs. Briggs in her hospital room, he came out and wrote three pages of notes on the encounter. (Tip: If you begin the sentence with a dependent clause, you should place a comma after that dependent clause. You should not use a comma if you begin the sentence with an independent clause.)

PRACTICE CORRECTING RUN-ONS

Use any of the four methods described to correct these run-ons.

1 Not all elderly patients are good historians those who have trouble giving their medical histories should bring a family member to medical appointments.

2 Dr. Rodman wrote an order for a chest x-ray for Mr. Smith 2 hours ago, however, the medical assistant from radiology has not arrived yet to pick Mr. Smith up.

3 James Albertson called to renew his asthma prescription, Dr. Babson wants James to come in for an examination before renewing the prescription.

4 Maria studied all night for her medical ethics final, she's still not sure she understands the debate on stem cell research.

5 Mr. Matwick arrived 25 minutes late for his neurology appointment Dr. Lowe was still able to see Mr. Matwick promptly.

Section 10-7 (To accompany Chapter 7, "Patient Education")

Fragments

A sentence must have a subject and a verb, and it must be a complete thought. A *fragment* is missing either a subject or a verb, or it is not a complete thought (that is, it cannot stand on its own as an independent clause). Sometimes writers use fragments intentionally for emphasis.

- I want you to get out of bed and get dressed. Now! (*Now* is a fragment, having neither a subject nor a verb.)
- John studies day and night for his genetics class. Really, all the time. (*Really, all the time* is a fragment, having neither a subject nor a verb.)

It is important to be able to identify fragments and know how to correct them. Be on the lookout for the following three kinds of fragments.

Leaving Out the Verb
A fragment may occur by leaving out a verb.

- **Fragment:** The pharmacy filling hundreds prescriptions every day. (*Filling* is a participle, describing the pharmacy; the subject, *pharmacy*, has no real verb.)
- **Complete Sentence:** The pharmacy fills hundreds of prescriptions every day. (*Fills* is the verb.)

Leaving Out the Subject
A fragment may occur also by leaving out the subject.

- **Fragment:** The pharmacy fills hundreds of prescriptions. *And delivers them every day.* (The verb *delivers* has no subject.)
- **Complete Sentence:** The pharmacy fills and delivers hundreds of prescriptions every day. (*Pharmacy* is the subject; *fills* and *delivers* are the verbs describing what it does.)
- **Complete Sentence:** The pharmacy fills hundreds of prescriptions every day. It also delivers those prescriptions. (*It*, a pronoun referring to the antecedent *pharmacy*, is the subject of the second sentence.)

Using Only a Dependent Clause
A dependent clause contains a subject and a verb, but it cannot stand alone. A dependent clause must be joined to an independent clause to form a complete sentence.

Tip: Dependent clauses always begin with a subordinating conjunction (*because, if, when, while*) or a relative pronoun (*who, which, that*).

- **Fragment:** Because the elderly patient appeared confused and frightened during the physical. (This group of words does have a subject *patient* and a verb *appeared,* but this is still a fragment. It is not a complete thought and cannot stand alone. The reader is left asking, *"What happened because the elderly patient appeared confused and frightened?")*

■ **Complete Sentence:** Because the elderly patient appeared confused and frightened during the physical, the doctor asked the patient's daughter to come into the examination room. (The dependent clause *Because the elderly patient appeared confused and frightened during the physical* is now connected to the independent clause *the doctor asked the patient's daughter to come into the examination room,* creating a complete sentence.)

■ **Complete Sentence:** The elderly patient appeared confused and frightened during the physical. (Dropping the subordinating conjunction **because** forms a complete sentence.)

PRACTICE WITH ┃ CORRECTING FRAGMENTS

Correct each of the fragments below. (Note: not all of the groups of words are fragments.)

1 Marta is still not prepared for her anatomy test. Despite the fact that she began studying last week.

2 When the nurse gave the little boy his flu shot, he began to cry. Really loud.

3 Mr. Ortiz brought his daughter with him to his cardiology appointment. To help translate during the examination.

4 Dr. Simpson wants Mrs. Donaldson to come back for a follow-up appointment in two weeks. After she has been seen by neurology.

5 Because the nutritionist hasn't spoken to Mr. Barnes yet. Mr. Barnes is not ready to be discharged.

Verb Tense Errors

Try to remain consistent when using verb tense. Do not change verbs from one tense to another unless you indicate a change in time. Be sure that the tense you are using always matches the time you are describing.

■ **Verb Tense Error:** When the doctor *came* into the examination room, the patient *asks* an important question.

■ **Correct Version:** When the doctor *came* into the examination room, the patient *asked* an important question.

■ **Verb Tense Error:** The nurse *spoke* to the patient about taking medicine regularly because the patient *will not be following* the directions on the prescription.

■ **Correct Version:** The nurse *spoke* to the patient about taking the medicine regularly because the patient *had not followed* the directions on the prescription.

- **Verb Tense Error:** The patient states that when he closes his eyes he feels dizzy. He closes his eyes yesterday afternoon at work and feels so dizzy he has to sit down and take a break. (The second sentence is describing a specific time in the past, so the sentence should use the past tense.)
- **Correct Version:** The patient states that when he closes his eyes he feels dizzy. He closed his eyes yesterday afternoon at work and felt so dizzy he had to sit down and take a break.

| PRACTICE WITH | TENSES |

Underline the correct tense of each verb in parentheses.

1 Yesterday Mr. Johnson (**calls/called**) to make an appointment for his physical examination.
2 Dr. Singh (**will be/has been**) out of the country until next Thursday. He has an opening at 3:30 p.m. on Friday.
3 When Dr. Gonzalez (**was/has been**) here last week, he renewed James's prescription for an asthma inhaler.
4 Janette (**works/has worked**) in this practice since 2002.
5 Before he finished school and passed his licensure exam, Jean (**works/had worked**) weekends as a unit clerk on the hematology ward.

Section 10-8 (To accompany Chapter 8, "Cultural Sensitivity in Healthcare Communication")

Paragraphing Basics

After the sentence, the most basic unit of writing is the paragraph. Writers use sentences to build paragraphs when describing or explaining ideas that are too complex to communicate with a single sentence. The length of paragraphs can vary, depending upon the complexity of the idea the writer wants to communicate. Readers can often identify paragraphs easily because the first line of any paragraph may be indented. As readers, we are trained early in our education to recognize paragraphs as essential units of communicating important ideas.

Paragraph Structure

Paragraphs generally use a structure that contains three elements: (1) the topic sentence, (2) supporting sentences, and (3) the concluding sentence.

Topic Sentence

The topic sentence is often the first sentence in the paragraph, and it expresses the paragraph's main idea.

Supporting Sentences

The supporting sentences of a paragraph provide the reader with the details that make up the main idea of the paragraph. Each supporting sentence explains some aspect of the idea in the topic sentence.

Concluding Sentence

Usually the final sentence in the paragraph, the concluding sentence, summarizes the ideas of the paragraph and provides a closing. The closing can be any of the following: a solution to the problem discussed in the paragraph, a prediction based on the elements described in the paragraph, a recommendation based on the facts presented in the paragraph, or a restatement of the main idea of the paragraph.

Examples of Paragraph Elements

Example 1

Topic Sentence: Effective communication skills are important in all of the healthcare professions.

Supporting Sentences: Good communication improves patient satisfaction, compliance, and healthcare outcomes. Professionals who can communicate effectively are better prepared to work with other members of the healthcare team.

Concluding Sentence: Hospitals, practices, and other healthcare organizations rightly value good communication skills as one of the most important strengths employees can have.

Complete Paragraph

Effective communication skills are important in all of the healthcare professions. Good communication improves patient satisfaction, compliance, and healthcare outcomes. Professionals who can communicate effectively are better prepared to work with other members of the healthcare team. Hospitals, practices, and other healthcare organizations rightly value good communication skills as one of the most important strengths employees can have.

Example 2

Topic Sentence: Heart attacks can occur most often because of a condition called coronary artery disease, or CAD.

Supporting Sentences: This disease involves is the buildup over many years of a fatty material, called plaque, on the inner walls of the coronary arteries. When such a buildup has occurred, a section of plaque can break open, causing a blood clot to form on the surface of the plaque.

Concluding Sentence: A heart attack occurs if the clot becomes large enough to cut off most or all of the blood flow to the part of the heart muscle fed by the artery.

Complete Paragraph: Heart attacks can occur most often because of a condition called coronary artery disease, or CAD. This disease involves is the buildup over many years of a fatty material, called plaque, on the inner walls of the coronary arteries. When such a buildup has occurred, a section of plaque can break open, causing a blood clot to form on the surface of the plaque. A heart attack occurs if the clot becomes large enough to cut off most or all of the blood flow to the part of the heart muscle fed by the artery.

PRACTICE WITH **PARAGRAPHS**

For the paragraphs below, identify the topic sentence (TS), the supporting sentences (SS), and the concluding sentence (CS).

1 While the flu and the common cold are both respiratory illnesses that have similar symptoms and may be difficult to distinguish, these two illnesses are caused by different viruses. The flu generally is worse than the common cold, and symptoms such as fever, body aches, extreme tiredness, and dry cough are more common and intense. Colds are usually milder than the flu. People with colds are more likely to have a runny or stuffy nose. Colds usually do not result in serious health problems, such as pneumonia, bacterial infections, or hospitalizations. Finally, the flu is caused by the influenza virus, which is a respiratory virus, whereas the common cold is caused by either the adenovirus or the corona virus, of which there are many different subsets.

2 A healthcare professional—any professional, for that matter—needs to have effective interpersonal skills. These are the skills one relies on most in order to have successful interaction with other people. These skills—which include tactfulness, courtesy, respect, empathy, genuineness, appropriate self-disclosure, and assertiveness—usually do not stand alone in isolation but rather exist in concert with each other. A healthcare professional who exhibits one of these skills as part of effective communication tends to exhibit others as well.

Section 10-9 (To accompany Chapter 9, "Electronic Communication")

The Basics of SOAP Notes

The most commonly used form of patient progress note is the SOAP note. Introduced in the late 1960s by Dr. Lawrence Weed, the SOAP

(Subjective-Objective-Assessment-Plan) note is a method for providing a logical and reproducible framework for generating medical records. Properly taken, SOAP notes allow healthcare professionals and organizations to transcribe and communicate patient encounters accurately, objectively, and effectively.

The SOAP note has four parts.

1 **S – Subjective.** This is the history and subjective information provided to the HCP by the patient or family member. For example, the patient may complain of feelings of nausea, chest pain, or headache.

2 **O – Objective.** This is the objective data from the HCP's examination of the patient. For example, the HCP may conduct a physical examination and detect that the patient has redness or inflammation, has difficulty breathing, or is hot to the touch. The HCP may also use vital signs or test results.

3 **A – Assessment.** This is the HCP's assessment (with diagnoses and impressions).

4 **P – Plan.** This is the patient's treatment plan, which may include prescriptions for medications, consults, surgery, or patient education.

Review Questions on SOAP
Choose the best answer.

1 _Pt. has chronic bronchitis_ is an example of
A) objective data based on the HCP's examination of the patient.
B) the HCP's assessment.
C) the patient's treatment plan.

2 _"I have a terrible stomach ache," the patient reports_ is an example of
A) subjective data from the patient.
B) the HCP's assessment.
C) the patient's treatment plan.

3 _Pt. will follow up with radiology in 2 weeks_ is an example of
A) the HCP's assessment.
B) the patient's treatment plan.
C) objective data based on the HCP's examination of the patient.

4 _V.S. taken: T-101, P-85, R-30, B.P. 140/80_ is an example of
A) subjective data from the patient.
B) objective data based on the HCP's examination of the patient.
C) the patient's treatment plan.

5 _PT complains of nausea and temperature_ is an example of
A) subjective data from the patient.
B) objective data based on the HCP's examination of the patient.
C) the HCP's assessment.

Acknowledgment of Receipt of Notice of Privacy Practices: a document to be signed by the patient acknowledging receipt of HIPAA privacy guidelines followed by healthcare providers

Acknowledgment: a statement of an occurrence, as in the acknowledgment of the receipt of an employee manual

Adherence: like "compliance," the act of following appropriate standards, procedures, or directions

Affect: a facial expression indicating any feeling or emotion, or the absence of feeling or emotion

Aggressiveness: a blaming, or attacking, of others to shield one's self or one's feelings

Ambiguous: open to more than one interpretation

Appropriate self-disclosure: the revealing of information about one's self or past at an appropriate time and place in any relationship

Assertiveness: a standing up for what one believes is right

Auditory learners: individuals who prefer to be engaged verbally with the use of questions and answers or discussion

Authoritative: having the quality of having greater rank, or authority

Body language: behaviors such as gestures, facial expressions, gaze patterns, positioning, posture, and touch that convey nonverbal messages to an observer

Candid: truthful and straightforward

Channel: the pathway or medium used to carry a message

Clarify: to make a message less confused and more clearly understandable

Closed body posture: a body position such as crossed arms and legs, leaning back, or turning the body away that creates distance between that individual and another

Closed question: a question designed to elicit a short, focused response such as a simple *yes* or *no*

Cognizant: being aware, knowing

Collaborator: a person who works with another to accomplish a task both want to accomplish

Commentary: comments or explanations of what is currently occurring

Communication: the successful transfer of a message and meaning from one person or group to another

Compensation: to overemphasize a trait or behavior in one area because of a belief that one must make up for a deficiency in another area

Compliance: like "adherence," the act of following appropriate standards, procedures, instructions, or directions

Comprehend: to understand

Congruent: fitting together, matching

Content: the subject matter of a message

Continuer: an expression designed to encourage an individual to reveal more information such as "*what else?*" or "*anything else?*"

Coping strategies: strategies for managing painful or difficult situations, thoughts, or feelings

Courtesy: a consideration for others' well-being, feelings, or needs

Cross-cultural: concerning, or moving between, cultures, as in "cross-cultural communication"

Cues: signs or indicators of a particular message

Cultural awareness: in the Campinha-Bacote model of cultural competence, the process of looking closely and honestly at your own biases toward other cultures, as well as examining your own cultural background. Cultural awareness includes an awareness that racism and other forms of discrimination exist in healthcare delivery

Cultural blindness: in the Georgetown University's Child Development Center's model, the stance taken by many people or institutions of viewing and treating all people from different cultures as if they were the same

Cultural competence: as defined by the American Medical Association, cultural competence is "the knowledge and interpersonal skills that allow providers to understand, appreciate, and work with individuals from cultures other than their own. It involves an awareness and acceptance of cultural differences; self-awareness; knowledge of the patient's culture; and adaptation of skills"; in the Georgetown University's Child Development Center's model, a term to describe individuals who or institutions that demonstrate an acceptance and respect for cultural differences

Cultural desire: in the Campinha-Bacote model of cultural competence, the all-important desire of the healthcare professional to become more culturally knowledgeable and skillful. It is important to emphasize that this has to be something the healthcare professional genuinely wants to do instead of merely a need to fulfill a job requirement

Cultural destructiveness: in the Georgetown University's Child Development Center's model, a stance characterized by attitudes, policies, structures, and practices by an individual or within a system or organization that are destructive to members of a cultural group

Cultural encounter: in the Campinha-Bacote model of cultural competence, the active seeking of face-to-face encounters with members of other cultures in order to better understand the HCP's own beliefs about other cultures and to prevent stereotyping

Cultural incapacity: in the Georgetown University's Child Development Center's model, the inability of an individual or institution to respond effectively to the needs and interests of culturally and linguistically diverse groups

Cultural knowledge: in the Campinha-Bacote model of cultural competence, the process of seeking a thorough understanding of the attitudes and beliefs of other cultural and ethnic groups, as well as the health conditions and diseases that exist among diverse ethnic groups

Cultural pre-competence: in the Georgetown University's Child Development Center's model, a term to describe the level of awareness by people or institutions of their capacity for growth in responding effectively to culturally and linguistically diverse groups

Cultural proficiency: in the Georgetown University's Child Development Center's model, a term to describe individuals or institutions that have a high regard for diverse culture and use this ethical stance as a foundation to guide their endeavors

Cultural skill: in the Campinha-Bacote model of cultural competence, the ability to accurately understand the cultural details surrounding the patient's presenting problem and to physically assess the patient within the context of their culture

Decode: to translate a message from its encoded form into a form the receiver understands

Defensiveness: a personalization of a response to any perceived criticism

Denial: to not admit the existence of specific circumstances (e.g., a cancer diagnosis or a disease's symptoms)

Diplomacy: a display of consideration in dealing with others' feelings or opinions

Directive tone: a tone of voice expressing authority and judgment, indicating a difference in professional rank

Disparity: a difference, usually a difference describing an inequality

Displacement: to avoid accepting ownership of one's thoughts, feelings, or desires and to direct them to someone or something else unrelated to their actual source

Dissociation: the disconnecting of emotions or feelings from the events or situations that caused the emotions or feelings

Elaborate: to add more detail to a message

Elicit: to draw or bring out, as in "to elicit an answer"

Email: an electronic message sent via computer

Emotion: a specific feeling, sentiment, or attitude

Empathic: indicating empathy

Empathy: the ability to understand what another person is feeling, virtually to the point of feeling what that person is feeling

Encode: to put the idea into some form that can be communicated as a message

Enunciate: to say or pronounce clearly

Ethnic: used to describe large groups of people who identify by common racial, national, tribal, linguistic, religious, or cultural origin

Ethnicity: an ethnic affiliation or identity

Expletives: swear words or curses

Express: to show feeling

Expressive tone: a tone of voice expressing emotion and feeling

Eye contact: looking at another individual in their eyes

Facial expression: a look on the face that conveys feeling or emotion

Facsimile, or FAX: an exact copy or reproduction of a document; a method of transmitting images or printed material by electronic means

Feedback: in the communication process, a response to the sender of a message

Figure of speech: a word or phrase used in a nonliteral sense to add force or effect to a message

Forthcoming: willing to divulge or provide information

Gaze pattern: a way of looking at another individual

Genuineness: the presenting to others of one's real, or true, self through words and actions

Gesture: a movement of a body part, especially the hands, to give an expression of feeling

Grief: a feeling of deep distress or sadness

HCP: Healthcare professional

Health literacy: the degree to which individuals have the capacity to obtain, process, and understand basic health information and services needed to make appropriate health decisions

Healthcare team: all of the people who work together in a healthcare organization to provide patient care

HIPAA Privacy Rule: also known as *The HIPAA Standards for Privacy of Individually Identifiable Health Information*, the federal law requiring healthcare organizations to protect patients' rights by ensuring the privacy of their health information

HIPAA: Health Insurance Portability and Accountability Act

Identification: to mimic the behavior or feelings of another person in order to conceal one's own natural behavior or feelings

Idiom: an expression that is unique to a group or language, the meaning of which is not understandable by the expression's literal meaning

Illustrator: a gesture used to emphasize, clarify, or add to the verbal content to a message; a gesture that shows how to do something

Infer: to reach a conclusion about a matter based on evidence you observe

Inhibit: to discourage or prevent from doing something

Innate: inborn, natural

Instructional context: refers to the environment in which the instruction will take place (e.g., doctor's office, hospital room, nursing home, outpatient clinic)

Interpersonal: any act, communication, or relationship between people

Interpret: to obtain meaning, to translate, to explain

Interviewee: the individual that is interviewed

Intimate distance: a distance of up to 1.5 feet between individuals

Jargon: highly technical language used by specialists

Kinesics: that which involves body movement in communication, such as gestures, facial expressions, and gaze patterns

Kinesthetic learners: individuals who learn by the physical demonstration of a task or technique by the HCP followed by the practice of the technique by the patient

Leading question: a question that prompts or encourages a desired answer

Leakage: the unintentional expression of feelings

Linguistic: having to do with languages

Listen: to hear with thoughtful attention or consideration

Literal: taking words at their usual or most basic sense

Medium: a means or channel for transferring a message

Message: a piece of communication containing information

Metaphor: a figure of speech in which a word or phrase is applied to an object or action which is not literal (e.g., his recovery from his injury was like climbing a mountain)

Minimizing a patient's feelings: to diminish, or make light of, a patient's feelings or emotions

Misinterpret: to obtain an incorrect meaning, to translate or explain incorrectly

Monitor: to assess

Multicultural: culturally diverse or having many different cultures, as in a society that is multicultural, or culturally diverse

Negative gesture: a body movement that is interpreted unfavorably by another individual

Noise: anything that disrupts or inhibits the communication process

Noncompliance: the act of not following appropriate standards, procedures, instructions, or direction

Nonjudgmental: unbiased, neutral, or unprejudiced in one's opinions

Nonverbal communication: communication through body movements, facial expressions, and gestures

Notice of Privacy Practices (NPP): a document provided by healthcare organizations to patients that states policies and procedures by which patient health information may be disclosed

Objective: not influenced by personal feelings or opinions

Open body posture: a body position such as uncrossed arms and legs and leaning forward that conveys a relaxed and approachable message

Open-ended question: a question designed to elicit a response that is elaborate and detailed; a question that may begin with *how* or *what*

Open-ended statement: a statement designed to elicit a response that is elaborate and detailed

Paraphrase: to use one's own words to repeat what someone else has said

Patient demographics: refer to certain characteristics of the patient that may influence their response to the instruction

Personal distance: a distance of 1.5 to 4 feet, or about an arm's length, between individuals

Personal space: the area or territory surrounding an individual in which they feel a sense of security and control

Pitch: the degree of highness or lowness of a voice or a tone

Plain language: language that an individual can understand the first time they hear it or read it

Position: the proximity and posture on an individual in relation to another

Positive gesture: body movement that is interpreted favorably by another individual

Posture: a type of body position that conveys feeling

Power dynamic: the hierarchical or authoritative relationship between individuals

Problem-solving tone: a tone of voice using reason, objectivity, and analysis

Professionalism: a manner of behavior appropriate to the allied healthcare workplace

Projection: to assign to another person or thing one's own feelings, thoughts, or desires

Proxemics: that which involves the physical distance between individuals when they communicate, such as territoriality and personal space, position, and posture

Prying: the pressuring of another to reveal information they might not otherwise reveal

Public distance: a distance of more than 12 feet between individuals

Rapport: in relationships, used to indicate harmony, empathy, sympathy, or trust

Rationalization: to use false reasoning to justify inappropriate or unacceptable behavior

Receiver: in the communication process, the person or group who receives and interprets a message

Regression: to unconsciously return to immature, or even infantile, behaviors or thoughts

Regulate: to control

Rephrase: express in an alternative way

Repression: to put out of one's mind painful or difficult thoughts, feelings, ideas, or events

Respect: to regard as worthy of special consideration

Roadblock to therapeutic communication: any obstruction or distraction that inhibits therapeutic communication

SOAP Notes: Subjective-Objective-Assessment-Plan note is a method for providing a logical and reproducible framework for generating medical records. Properly taken, SOAP notes allow for healthcare professionals and organizations to transcribe and communicate patient encounters accurately, objectively, and effectively

Self-disclosure: the revealing of information about one's self or one's past

Sender: the person or group who initiates the communication process

Shorthand: a simpler, shorter way of communicating

Simile: a figure of speech involving the comparison of one thing and another thing of a different kind (e.g., he is as sick as a dog)

Situational context: refers to the medical condition that creates the need for the instruction

Slang: a form of language that consists of words or phrases that are considered very informal and are typically associated with a particular group

Small talk: talk about everyday events and occurrences, intended to fill time

Social distance: a distance of 4 to 12 feet between individuals

Standard English: English in its most widely accepted form, as written and spoken by educated people, both formally and informally

Subjective: influenced by personal feelings or opinions

Tactfulness: consideration in dealing with others' feelings or opinions

Teach back: when an individual repeats information or instructions in their own words

Telecommunication: communication via telephone

Tenor: in a relationship, the mood or condition

Therapeutic communication: communication between the HCP and patient that pertains to the patient's well-being and care

Therapeutic relationship: the relationship between the HCP and the patient, the purpose of which is to advance the patient's well-being and care

Tone of voice: a way of speaking that conveys feeling or the tenor of a relationship

TPO: abbreviation for "treatment, payment, and healthcare operations"

Trait: a characteristic or tendency

Transmit: to send information

Universal: that which is everywhere, which affects everyone

Verbal communication: communication using words

Verbalize: to express in words

Visual learners: individuals who respond well to the use of pictures, diagrams, anatomicmodels, and literature

White coat syndrome: a term to describe a patient's behavior when in the presence of an HCP, often indicating an increased level of patient compliance or, perhaps, anxiety because of the presence of the HCP